This book is a timely, practihose
aspiring to or currently engag   nent.
Dr. Robinson has more than   ging
health projects worldwide, an   tical
experience and lessons he gair   ding
to evaluation, all critical aspect   ⌐ here
in a practical and straightforward manner.

Henry B. Perry, MD, PhD, MPH, *Senior Associate,*
Department of International Health, Johns Hopkins
Bloomberg School of Public Health, USA

Using numerous examples and case studies, this novel practical hand-
book guides us through all phases of public health project management,
from theory to operations and practice. It highlights how successful
global health projects interact deeply with local communities and stakeholders, working with multiple sectors and international and local partners in LMICs.

Steven Ault, MSc, MRSB, REHS, FRSTMH, PAHO/WHO
Senior Advisor, Neglected Infectious Diseases (retired), Adjunct
Lecturer, School of Public Health, University of Maryland, USA

'Managing Global Health Projects in LMICs' captures all the critical
stages of project management cycle while providing a concrete lens on
the realities, challenges, and problem-solving methods that guarantee
effective and high impact results. Dr. Robinson has deep knowledge and
experience working in such contexts, thus providing very practical case
studies and contextual examples that enable readers to engage in 'real
world' learning.

Ann Canavan, BA, RN, MSc, MPH, *Senior Director,*
International Medical Corps, Switzerland

Managing Global Health Projects in Low and Middle-Income Countries

With over 30 years of experience in global health programming and teaching, the author offers practical and insightful guidance in this unique book for managing global health projects in resource-constrained settings.

Beginning with an overview of fundamental principles, the book delves deeply into a 'nuts and bolts' approach to health project management. From building project teams and developing detailed activity plans to evaluating health projects and report writing, this book brings the readers a wealth of knowledge they can use to manage health projects. Besides a list of key takeaways and discussion questions, each chapter features a case study exercise from real life situation where readers can picture themselves as project managers, sharpening their understanding of concepts and strategies.

Timely and original, this book is an essential resource for university students of global health courses preparing to manage global health projects in low- and middle-income countries, as well as for newly engaged project managers.

Dr. Paul Robinson is a physician and global health professional with over three decades of international experience in global health programming. He has managed health programs; developed program proposals, partnerships, and reports; mentored and trained staff; and directed technical teams in low- and middle-income countries and in organizational headquarters in the US. He has worked with several non-government, non-profit, and UN organizations. He taught university course on global health as an adjunct professor.

Managing Global Health Projects in Low and Middle-Income Countries
A Practical Guide

Paul Robinson

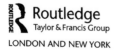
Routledge
Taylor & Francis Group

LONDON AND NEW YORK

Designed cover image: Getty Images

First published 2024
by Routledge
4 Park Square, Milton Park, Abingdon, Oxon OX14 4RN

and by Routledge
605 Third Avenue, New York, NY 10158

Routledge is an imprint of the Taylor & Francis Group, an informa business

British Library Cataloguing-in-Publication Data
A catalogue record for this book is available from the British Library

ISBN: [978-1-032-52105-3] (hbk)
ISBN: [978-1-032-50588-6] (pbk)
ISBN: [978-1-003-40524-5] (ebk)

DOI: 10.4324/9781003405245

Typeset in Sabon
by KnowledgeWorks Global Ltd.

Dedication

To my wife, Pronoti:

Thank you for your inspiration and support that made the writing of this book possible.

Contents

Author biography

Dr. Paul Robinson is a physician and public health professional with over 30 years of international experience in Global Health programming. His responsibilities included:

- Technical management of health programs in Maternal Newborn and Child Health, Child Survival, Reproductive Health, HIV/AIDS, tuberculosis, and Supply Chain Management of health commodities.
- Developing program partnerships, proposals, reports, and presentations.
- Mentoring and training staff.

His work experience includes senior positions with CARE International, Plan International, American Red Cross, John Snow Inc., UNICEF, International Medical Corps, Action Against Hunger, and Northrup-Grumman's Global AIDS program.

Dr. Robinson has taught graduate-level course on global health at the School of Public Health at the University of Maryland, USA, as Adjunct Professor.

He has a Medical Degree (MBBS) from Chittagong Medical College in Chittagong, Bangladesh, and a Master's Degree in Public Health (MPH) from the Johns Hopkins University Bloomberg School of Public Health in Baltimore, Maryland, USA. He has also done post-doctoral studies at JHU/SPH. He holds a Master's Degree in theology from Cornerstone Theological Seminary in Grand Rapids, Michigan, USA.

Dr. Robinson has traveled to and provided technical assistance in over twenty-five countries in Africa, the Caribbean, Latin America, South Asia, and the former Soviet Union.

He is a Global Health consultant based in Florida, USA.

List of abbreviations

ANC	Antenatal care
AOB	Any Other Business
APM	Assistant project manager
BvA	Budget vs. actual
CBO	Community Based Organization
CDC	Community development committee
CHC	Community health committee
CHP	Community health promoters
CHV	Community health volunteer
CHW	Community health worker
CV	Curriculum Vitae
DAP	Detailed Activity Plan
EPI	Expanded Program on Immunization
EVD	Ebola virus disease
FBO	Faith Based Organization
FGD	Focus Group Discussion
HC	Health center
HR	Human resources
ICCM	Integrated Community Case Management
ICRC	International Committee of the Red Cross
IFRC	International Red Cross and Red Crescent Movement
KII	Key Informant Interview
LLIN	Long-lasting insecticide-treated net
LMIC	Low- and middle-income country
LT	Laboratory Technician
MEAL	Monitoring Evaluation Accountability and Learning
MNCH	Maternal newborn and child health
MOH	Ministry of Health
MPH	Master in Public Health
MSF	Médecins Sans Frontières
MUAC	Mid-upper arm circumference
NGO	Non-government organization

OJT	On-the-job training
ORS	Oral Rehydration Salt
PM	Project manager
PO	Project officer
RDT	Rapid diagnostic test kit
ROM	Rough order of magnitude
SMART	Specific, Measurable, Achievable, Relevant, and Time-bound
STEM	Support, Train, and Empower Managers
TB	Tuberculosis
TC	Training Coordinators
UNDP	United Nations Development Program
UNHCR	United Nations High Commissioner for Refugees
UNICEF	United Nations Children's Fund
VDC	Village development committee
VHC	Village health committee
WFP	UN World Food Program
WHO	World Health Organization

List of figures, images and tables

Figures

Images

Tables

A message from the author to the reader

Greetings!

If you have picked up this book in your hands and are reading this page, you could be a student pursuing a postgraduate course in public health such as the Master in Public Health (MPH) or a similar degree. You may be aspiring to become a project manager (PM) for leading a global public health project in a low- and middle-income country (LMIC) following your graduation. Alternatively, you may already be a PM placed in a resource constraint setting with the role of managing a global health project in an LMIC. Perhaps, you are preparing to function as a project advisor or specialist based in an organization's regional office or headquarters and often traveling to project countries and sites to support global health teams. If any of these descriptions fits you, this book will be immensely valuable to you.

How do I know that? You see, three decades ago I was where you are today ... a student at a prestigious university in the United States, completing my MPH degree course. Following my graduation I went to a resource constraint country in South Asia, where I suddenly found myself managing a large global health project, with more than two hundred project staff in my team.

I quickly realized I had learned quite well the *principles* of global health programming in the classrooms of my university. Now, however, I had to quickly learn the practical *'how to'*s of managing such a large project that covered one-fourth of the country. It was the *practical application* of the theoretical knowledge that became extremely critical in managing this large project. And which I needed to master rapidly in the field, stumbling through successes and failures.

To give you a few examples, as a fresh graduate I knew the importance of systematically educating the village mothers about the need to immunize their children with vaccines. But I lacked the know-how of mobilizing a large project team to ensure community health workers were using proper teaching materials in vaccine education sessions. I needed to learn how to train my project staff in a timely manner so they could organize these sessions effectively. I had to quickly find ways to make sure the nurses and the vaccinators had enough vaccines stored at the correct temperature in the rural health centers. Again, I knew the communities needed to use bed nets to prevent malaria but had to learn how to budget for these bed nets, how to procure and store enough of these nets well ahead of the distribution, and to oversee the actual distribution of the bed nets among community members. And so on ...

Later in my career as the PM for several other global health projects in a number of LMICs it was my responsibility to select staff, train them, supervise them, and inspire them. I needed to make sure my projects had detailed activity plans, which the project teams would follow. It was my role to develop and track project budgets, arrange for project evaluations, write project reports, and make presentations to internal and external audiences.

Further down the career lane, I was based at several organizational headquarters in the USA from where I would travel around the world to support global health projects in LMICs. Serving as a technical specialist, health project advisor, director of technical units, and consultant, I needed to provide support to PMs and their teams in more than twenty-five countries.

There was no book that I could read and quickly study the details of how teams were supposed to conduct key project activities. Or how to manage global health project teams. Over the years, I had to learn all this the hard way – observing, experimenting, sometimes failing, and then succeeding, brainstorming with others, and learning from experience, updating myself with recent publications, and so forth. Looking back, I wish I had a textbook that would tell me in a practical way how to actually *manage* and *lead* a global health project.

Years later I taught graduate students at a university in the United States a course on global health program management and evaluation. Again, when I looked around for a textbook to recommend to my students, I found none that would give them *practical*, 'nuts and bolts' guidance on how to set up and run global health projects.

Well, *this* book comes to you as that missing guide. A practical manual that will prepare you to manage a global health project when you are placed in a resource constraint setting in an LMIC. I have authored this book based on my own experience and the experience of others whom I have closely observed and worked with as I journeyed on my career path in several countries of Asia, Africa, the Caribbean, Eastern Europe, and Latin America.

Whether you are a global health graduate student at a university, a health project manager in an LMIC, or serving as a specialist or advisor at your organization's headquarters, you will find in the pages that follow, three decades of experience consolidated just for you ... from someone who once was in your shoes.

As you study this book you could be preparing for a rewarding career that will have a profound impact. You have the potential to make a significant difference in the lives of many families and communities in resource constraint settings. However, there may be times when the challenges will seem insurmountable, and you may want to give up. Fear not – this book offers several ways to equip you for those challenges and encourages you to persevere.

I wish you the very best as you study this book and prepare to become a leader in global health.

Thank you for reading!

Dr. Paul Robinson, MBBS, MPH, MTS.

Introduction

Purpose of the book

Dr. Paul Robinson, a medical doctor and global health professional, writes this book from his own experience and from that of others about how to manage projects designed to improve the health of communities in Low- and Middle-Income Countries (LMICs). These management functions include building health project teams, developing detailed project work plans, increasing staff capacity, supervising project staff, communicating with project teams, interacting with external stakeholders, managing project budgets, monitoring and evaluating health projects, and reporting project progress, among others. Dr. Robinson gives practical information and ideas on these key aspects of global health project management.

You will find in these chapters clear and pragmatic instructions and examples to help you carry out your essential management functions when you prepare to assume the role of a global health project manager (PM). Although written for those that are preparing to manage global health projects in LMICs a significant part of the book's content also can be applied to the management of non-health projects. This is because there is much common ground in project management roles and practices in both health and non-health environments.

How to use the book

The book serves an important purpose in the global health education field by filling a critical gap in existing publications. It is primarily intended to be used as a textbook for graduate students seeking to become proficient in managing health projects in LMICs and preparing to become PMs, health program advisors, and leaders.

Also, there is very little literature available today that adequately tells a PM who has been recently placed in the field in an LMIC, what exactly needs to be done to manage a global health project. The pages that

DOI: 10.4324/9781003405245-1

follow can serve as a valuable 'nuts and bolts' field guide for practicing professionals as well, especially those that are new in their project management role who need clear instructions and advice on how to manage global health projects. It provides a wealth of information that can help them lead teams and bring health and well-being to marginalized communities.

Features of the book

This book contains 11 chapters plus an introduction and a conclusion (Some final thoughts) – Chapter 12 – covering all the essential responsibilities that come with being a PM. Each chapter focuses on a specific function of the PM's role and ends with a summary list of *Key takeaways* to help you remember the important points of the chapter. *Discussion questions* are also included at the end of each chapter, which can be used as self-check tests to enable you to measure your learning, in small group brainstorming discussions, or for instructor-assisted discourse in the larger classroom setting. Additionally, each chapter features a *Case study exercise* reflecting a real-life scenario related to a management issue for you to find practical solutions. Attempt to solve these issues during your individual study and review time. Then share your solutions in small group discussions and larger classroom settings. The author's suggestions for these exercises are included at the back of the book. By going through these *Key takeaways*, *Discussion questions*, and *Case study exercises*, you will gain a more thorough understanding of the topics covered in each chapter and reinforce your learning.

Tone of the book

If you are a student of global health who aspires to lead project teams in LMICs this book encourages you to imagine yourself in the role of a PM and presents information as if you are already in this position. By placing yourself in the PM's shoes and learning about the PM's functions in each chapter, you can better prepare for a career in managing global health projects, and advising junior PMs. If you are currently employed as a PM for a global health project, you will find the tone of this book resonates with you as well.

In the PM role, you could work as a government Ministry of Health (MOH) staff or be employed by a local or international non-government organization (NGO) and stationed in the capital city or another town within the LMIC, where the global health project operates. Regardless of who your employer is, your job entails managing a team of trained global health professionals.

You will find the book's tone particularly refers to the PM who is recruited by an NGO. This is because, if you are pursuing an academic degree in a university located in the West or the Global North, the probability of your being recruited by an NGO in the West and placed in an LMIC in the Global South is high. Also, NGOs appear to possess the capacity to effectively develop and adapt their global health initiatives, significantly influencing how the MOH operates government health projects in many LMICs. With that being said, the author recognizes that you may decide to join the MOH in an LMIC to become a PM of a government global health project upon completing your studies. The book is useful for both types of PMs, irrespective of whether they work for the MOH or for an NGO.

In spite of the employer, being at the helm of your project is an enormous responsibility. The book provides a systematic guide to help you fulfill your duties as a successful PM. These tasks are both rewarding and exhilarating, bringing you a sense of satisfaction and accomplishment.

Terminologies used in this book

The PM leads a group of individuals. In this book, the terms 'team,' 'teammates,' 'team members,' 'supervisee,' and 'staff' are all used interchangeably to refer to this group.

Likewise, 'activities' and 'tasks' are the same describing the various functions of your project teammates. 'Sub-activities' and 'sub-tasks' are also equivalent terms.

In the context of funding your global health project, a 'donor' or 'donor agency/organization' is the same as a 'funding body/organization.' They provide the necessary financial support for project operations.

Typically, a project team has staff in various positions including those that supervise junior staff. For instance, assistant project managers have many administrative tasks to do, but also supervises junior staff that report to them. In that sense, they are 'supervisors.' Similarly, project officers supervise junior staff and volunteers, besides engaging in other activities. When it comes to project monitoring the term 'supervisor' and 'monitor' are sometimes used interchangeably. Supervisors that perform project monitoring are usually the project team members that have supervisory roles over junior staff.

As you have noted earlier, the PM is normally recruited by an organization (NGO or MOH) to manage its project in the field. This organization, which operates the project utilizing resources that it secures, is the 'implementing organization/agency.' The PM reports to their superiors within their implementing agency.

The term, 'LMIC' is based on the country classification used by the World Bank, where it stands for 'Lower Middle-Income Country.'[1] The World Bank also uses the term '<u>Low-</u> and Middle-Income Country' in its publications.[2] In this book 'LMIC' means <u>Low-</u> *and* Middle-Income countries. Global health projects operate in both low-income and middle-income countries of the world. This book is relevant to both contexts. LMICs are often in resource-constrained settings.

The author sincerely hopes that as you read and apply the guidelines in this book, you will discover them to be pragmatic and beneficial in your preparation for your PM role in global health.

Happy reading!

Notes

1 "World Bank Country and Lending Groups," accessed June 29, 2023, https://datahelpdesk.worldbank.org/knowledgebase/articles/906519
2 "Low & middle income," accessed June 29, 2003, https://data.worldbank.org/country/XO

References

The World Bank | Data. "Low & middle income." Accessed June 29, 2023. https://data.worldbank.org/country/XO

The World Bank | Working for a World Free of Poverty. "World Bank Country and Lending Groups." Accessed June 29, 2023.
https://datahelpdesk.worldbank.org/knowledgebase/articles/906519

1 The fundamentals of managing global health projects

In this chapter we will explore the fundamental practices of managing global health projects in LMICs. The chapter aims to provide answers to questions like, "What is the PM's role in leading and organizing their team's activities when carrying out global health projects?" and "What are some skills that the PM should develop for leading their team as they achieve project goals?" While the subsequent chapters will delve deeper into these and other topics, this chapter provides an overview of the key components of global health project management. However, before discussing project *management*, it is important to understand what we mean by a "project" and the unique characteristics of global health projects.

Global health projects

The health and well-being of citizens are typically the responsibility of the government of a country. The health care system is managed and designed primarily by the government's MOH. To promote the health of communities, various organizations create, develop, and implement health projects. These organizations may be the MOH, or NGOs that are for-profit contractors, or non-profit voluntary organizations. A team of trained health workers led by a PM implements health projects under the MOH or NGOs. Usually, NGOs carry out global health projects in LMICs where local resources are scarce, and the government requests their support. These NGO projects assist the MOH in providing preventive and curative health services to local communities.

The PM is normally based in the capital of the LMIC, or a large city where the project operates and reports to their superiors in their country office. In the case of a government project, the PM answers to a supervisor within the MOH. For example, the PM that leads a government malaria control project would ordinarily work under the malaria control division chief of the MOH.

DOI: 10.4324/9781003405245-2

This book focuses mainly on the operational functions of global health projects carried out by NGOs. However, many of these functions apply equally to the projects undertaken by the MOH. Regardless of whether implemented by the MOH or an NGO, all projects have the following common elements: *input, process, output,* and *outcome.* These elements define the project type, whether the project is a maternal health project or a malaria control project. Whether it is an HIV/AIDS project or a project that improves the health of young children, to give some examples.

Project elements

- Input. Like any other project, global health projects require resources to operate properly. These resources include project staff, funding, vehicles, office space, equipment, and other necessary items. Without these inputs, projects cannot function efficiently. In LMICs, global health projects are run by technical and administrative staff that the implementing organizations (both the MOH and NGOs) recruit. Funding is typically acquired through awards granted by funding agencies to these organizations. The MOH in some cases may have its own internal funding from sources other than the donor agencies.

- Process. The project process refers to the *implementation* of project activities using the available inputs. For instance, organizing health education sessions for village mothers to help them learn how to prepare Oral Rehydration Salt (ORS) solutions, training health center midwives to manage post-partum hemorrhage, and supplying rural dispensaries with essential medicines are some project activities. When undertaken in a systematic manner these activities contribute to the improvement of the health of the community members. This organized and systematic execution of the activities is known as the project process.

- Output. The process (project activities functioning together) produces certain *immediate* results. To continue with the examples given above, imagine that over the course of a month, a hundred village mothers attended education sessions on ORS preparation that the project organized. These hundred mothers constitute the project's output for that particular health education activity. Similarly, the number of midwives that attended the training session on post-partum hemorrhage management over one month, and the number of dispensaries that the project supplied with essential medicines over the same period are all examples of outputs for those respective project activities in that month. These are the direct and immediate results of the project processes.

- Outcome. When the direct outputs of the project produce benefits to the community it is called the project outcome. The outcomes are the positive *changes* that occur in the community because of the project's processes and outputs. Consider the same three examples from before. Suppose several children received ORS from the village mothers that attended the project's health education session on ORS preparation. As a result, the children did not have dehydration, which would have caused them to suffer or even die if they had not received the ORS. Also, a number of pregnant women received adequate management of post-partum hemorrhage at the time of their delivery from the midwives that the project trained. Furthermore, the dispensaries were able to avoid stockouts and provide essential medicines to patients because the project had supplied them with these medicines. These benefits in the community are the positive changes that the project has brought about. These are the project outcomes.

  Note that the outcomes are not immediate or direct results of the project processes involved. Outcomes are *indirect* results of project activities, and due to the time it takes to achieve them, they are not as immediately visible as the outputs.

  Figure 1.1 illustrates these four elements with a coffee maker. To prepare coffee the machine needs dry coffee powder or beans and water, which are the INPUTS. By utilizing these resources, the coffee maker grinds, mixes, heats, filters, and delivers its immediate

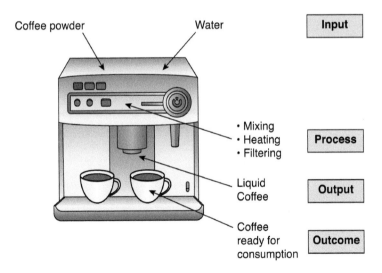

Figure 1.1 Project input, process, output, and outcome

product – liquid coffee. The grinding or mixing, heating, and filtering together constitute the PROCESS of the coffee maker. Through this process, the machine produces freshly brewed liquid coffee, which is its direct and immediate OUTPUT. When served in a cup, this coffee provides a stimulating beverage that benefits the consumer. For coffee lovers, this drink brings about a refreshing change, a benefit, which is the OUTCOME of the coffee maker's process and output.

- Impact. The impact of a project is an important element that we will touch on briefly. It refers to the higher level long-term benefits that a health project provides to the population it serves. For instance, a project can lead to a reduction in death rates in young children from dehydration. However, it is worth noting that a single health project may not necessarily cause a significant reduction in morbidity and mortality rates. Other factors such as women's education and their income generation, better agricultural yields, and a stronger healthcare system can also indirectly impact these rates. As a result, impact is rarely prioritized or measured as an indicator of a single project's success. In this book, impact is not highlighted as a key project element, since global health projects only *contribute* to the attaining of these higher level achievements (impacts), but do not directly cause them.

Project Characteristics

Like any other projects, global health initiatives have distinct characteristics.

- Each project is unique, with its own set of inputs, processes, outputs, and outcomes.
- Projects are temporary and have a defined start and end date. They end when they have achieved their planned goals and objectives or can no longer continue due to various reasons.
- Success is measured not only by meeting goals but also by fulfilling stakeholder expectations. Key stakeholders include the project communities, MOH, donor agencies, and the implementing organization.

Project phases

Global health projects typically run through four basic phases during their life cycle, which can somewhat overlap with each other. Figure 1.2 illustrates these four cyclical phases of a project life.

- Planning phase. The first phase is the planning phase, which involves developing a detailed project proposal that outlines its inputs, processes, outputs, and outcomes. As the PM you may step into this

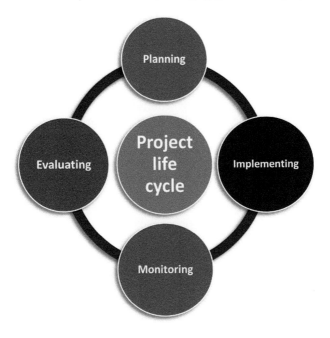

Figure 1.2 Global health project life cycle

phase when planning is already underway, or when your implementing organization has already submitted the project proposal to the funding agency. Alternatively, you may replace an outgoing PM and join the project team midway in its life cycle.

Once your project receives funding and you join the project team as its PM, you will need a copy of the project proposal, which outlines the plan and the budget for the project. The proposal has been approved by both the donor agency and your organization's senior management when you join the project. However, you will still need to fine-tune the proposal and develop a Detailed Activity Plan (DAP) with your project team. This detailed planning usually happens shortly after a project begins. The details of the DAP process are covered in Chapter 3.

- Implementing phase. During project implementation, the DAP is put into action. The PM oversees all the tasks and sub-tasks that the team performs and provides support to ensure work is done according to this plan. The PM spends most time and effort in this phase of the project maintaining communications by holding regular team meetings and individual meetings, visiting project sites, interacting with both internal and external stakeholders, and reviewing routine reports from the project's site managers to identify any deviations from the plan. If there are delays in project activities the PM takes corrective steps to bring the project back on track. If that fails, the PM modifies the plan and maintains detailed records of the variance, the reasons for deviation, and the way the plan was modified. The PM submits monthly or quarterly reports to project stakeholders and includes in these reports the deviations that occurred, and the changes made in the plan along with any corrective actions taken. The book covers a range of project implementation topics such as communications, interactions, reporting on variance, and more throughout the various chapters that follow.

- Monitoring phase. Project monitoring is an ongoing process that takes place throughout the project's entire life cycle. Chapter 9 provides a detailed discussion on monitoring. Specially trained members of the Monitoring Evaluation Accountability and Learning (MEAL) Team that belongs to the implementing organization set up computerized monitoring systems for projects and assist the PM in tracking project progress and reporting. These MEAL team colleagues may be in the country office where the PM is based, in regional offices, or in the organization's headquarters. They also provide support to the project by conducting periodic evaluations, which are discussed in Chapter 10.

- Evaluating phase. Throughout its life cycle, a health project is typically evaluated three times. A *baseline* evaluation takes place at the initiation of the project. A *mid-term* evaluation is then conducted at the halfway point, followed by a *final* evaluation upon completion of the project. Sometimes a project may need a special evaluation in certain situations (e.g., for evaluating an add on research initiative within the project, or a repeat evaluation if needed), but usually, the baseline, mid-term, and final evaluations are the three main ones. The PM can count on the MEAL Team to help in conducting evaluations.

  Evaluations – particularly the final evaluation – can often generate findings and insights which can inform the development of a future project as an extension of the current one. In this way the findings from the final evaluation become essential building blocks for the planning phase of the next round of the project, thus completing the current project's life cycle. Or the final evaluation may lead to the replication of the current project in a different geographical location.

These four phases of a project may not always occur in a strictly linear progression, as there can be some overlap between them. For instance, the monitoring of activities and the mid-term evaluation occur simultaneously with project implementation.

Project team structure

Global health projects are operated by teams of people who share a common health goal and common objectives. These objectives are determined by community needs. Each member of a project team contributes, in accordance with his or her competence and skill in coordination with the functions of others. Total Engagement of All Members of your project TEAM is a must for the global health project to be successful. Besides the management and technical staff, a global health project team can also include the support staff.[1]

There are various types of health project teams that are created based on the type of interventions they carry out and the activities they perform. Examples of interventions include nutrition, maternal newborn and child health (MNCH), reproductive health, HIV/AIDS, and tuberculosis (TB) control, and water and sanitation. Every intervention will have its own activities. For instance, the MNCH intervention involves a range of activities, such as providing antenatal care (ANC) services to pregnant women, training midwives on safe delivery and newborn care, administering routine immunization to children, educating community health workers (CHWs) on Integrated Community Case Management (ICCM), and supplying essential medicines to health centers. To achieve the project objective for each intervention, there must be a team with individuals trained in these various activities.

Thus, different types of projects may have different team structures. For example, some projects consist of a solitary intervention with a sizable team, which is then divided into sub-teams that handle distinct activities under that intervention. A global health project with one large team can be focused on a single intervention such as child immunization. The sub-teams within this large team might focus on separate areas such as training health workers on vaccinating children, supporting cold chain systems for vaccines, and improving health seeking behavior in the community so more caregivers would get their children vaccinated. Alternatively, other complex projects may have multiple interventions that are managed by one team, with each sub-team undertaking the activities of their corresponding intervention. An MNCH project would have a maternal health, a newborn health, and a child health intervention. Each of these three interventions would have its own set of activities and sub-activities, managed by three sub-teams.

The PM ensures the health project team composition matches the team function. In other words, you must have in your team those individuals that have the skills and experiences which allow them to conduct the team activities properly.

Global health project teams can be broadly categorized as those that are focused on the *demand* side and those on the *supply* side. The former work towards social mobilization and community participation to encourage better health practices at individual, family and community levels and create demand for quality health services. On the other hand, the latter support the provision of direct healthcare services, such as those offered in health centers.

To distinguish between the demand and supply side strategies consider community mothers voluntarily opting (i.e., demanding) for their children to get routine immunization instead of neglecting or avoiding it, which is what they used to do before the start of the project. This shift in practice is an example of a behavior change brought about by *demand-side* efforts of the project. Project workers through health education and related efforts influenced the mothers to switch from avoiding to adopting.

As an example of *supply-side* efforts skilled health workers at health facilities are providing adequate ANC services to pregnant women because your project has trained the facility staff on these services. You would want to ensure you have the appropriate types of skilled team members who can support either the demand side or the supply side activities or both in your project communities, depending on your project objectives and interventions.

During my early years managing global health projects, I was tasked with leading a child health project that focused solely on demand side intervention. Our focus was to encourage positive health behavior among women caregivers of young children in a rural area of Bangladesh. Through various activities, we were able to achieve success in several areas, such as promoting hand washing, providing adequate ORS to children with diarrhea and dehydration, using mosquito bed nets, and practicing birth spacing with modern contraceptives. To achieve these outcomes, I assembled a project team with members who possessed the necessary training and skills to execute each of these different tasks effectively.

Later in my career, I oversaw projects that solely focused on supply side interventions. In one such project, we provided support to rural health centers in Nagorno Karabakh – a small, disputed territory between Armenia and Azerbaijan – by reconstructing health center structures, supplying medicine and equipment, and training healthcare staff to care for patients.

As my career progressed, I continued to advise PMs and their teams on complex projects that required both demand and supply side interventions in several LMICs. Through all these experiences, I recognized how crucial it is to build project teams with skilled and trained individuals who can execute tasks and sub-tasks efficiently to achieve the desired project outcomes.

Basics of global health project management

As previously mentioned, global health project teams consist of a group of proficient individuals who collaborate and coordinate their efforts to attain the health project's objectives, goals, and outcomes.[2] To effectively manage such projects, the PM must *plan, organize, lead,* and *control* the human and other resources available for achieving the desired project goals, objectives, and outcomes. Traditionally these have been considered the four central functions of the PM.

Recently, however, there has been a shift toward the belief that project management should also prioritize *leadership* skills. This includes setting a clear vision and goals for the project team, effectively communicating these goals, and guiding team members toward achieving them. This viewpoint emphasizes that the PM should be more facilitative, participative, and empowering in the establishment and execution of their visions and goals. However, this does not necessarily entail a complete overhaul of the four primary management functions but rather a re-emphasis on the leadership aspects of management.[3] In the following discussion, we will still focus on these four cardinal functions while also highlighting the importance of visioning by PMs for their teams in a participatory and empowering manner.

Planning

Once your project proposal has been approved by the donor agency and senior management of your organization, it becomes the guiding plan for your project. However, this plan normally does not give detailed information on project activities. Therefore, it is critical to develop a more comprehensive plan, such as the DAP, as mentioned above. The DAP gives a more detailed schedule for accomplishing the tasks and sub-tasks for your project team.

For instance, if your proposal includes an intervention for HIV control, it might list key activities such as promoting condom use, educating on male circumcision, introducing rapid HIV tests, and supporting patients for treatment adherence. The DAP on the other hand will elaborate on each of these activities, for example giving information about when and how the project team will hold education sessions for promoting condom use and encouraging male circumcision, and the details of how rapid HIV tests will take place, as well as what the project will do to increase patients' treatment adherence. These are all activities under the HIV intervention.

During project implementation, it is necessary to plan the *exact* schedules and sites for different activities. To use the example of organizing education sessions, there must be plans for holding these educational sessions on a daily or weekly basis. Additionally, plans must be developed for preparing or procuring educational materials, organizing transport for those traveling to the sites to give education, selecting the venues for the sessions, arranging per diem for team members who will travel, and so on. This level of micro-planning for all the tasks and sub-tasks is more detailed than what is included in the proposal but is necessary for the day-to-day operation of the project. The PM does not plan the DAP and execute all the activities alone but has the support of the project team and even others that may be outside the team (e.g., logisticians, finance, and human resources colleagues) who provide assistance.

To prevent any potential misunderstandings or conflicts within the team, it is crucial to ensure that all individuals involved in undertaking the tasks and sub-tasks are well-informed of the detailed project plans and capable of executing them.

Organizing

In a project team, the PM is responsible for establishing structures that define the working and reporting relationships between team members. Sometimes this may involve organizing team members into sub-teams based on their respective tasks, as mentioned earlier. For instance, a sub-team may be needed to run mobile clinics that treat patients under a tent in a refugee camp setting as seen in Image 1.1, while another sub-team may coordinate health education for behavior change at the same or different location, as seen in Image 1.2.

The PM ensures that there are clear supervisory and reporting structures for each sub-team, and communicates these arrangements to all team members in a transparent manner.

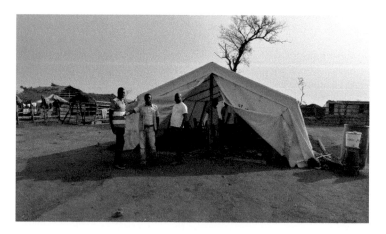

Image 1.1 Mobile health team at a refugee camp in Central African Republic

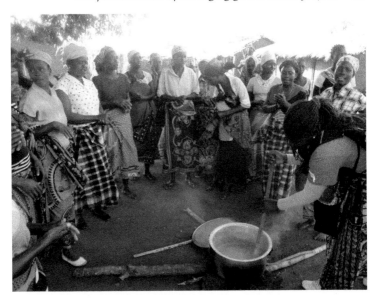

Image 1.2 Health project staff demonstrating to village women how to prepare nutritious food in rural Mozambique

Leading

The PM needs to develop a clear vision of how the project should operate to align with the organization's strategic goals. The PM empowers and inspires the project team to understand their individual roles in achieving the project objectives. Effective leadership requires the PM to leverage their position, personality, influence, communication style, and persuasive skills to motivate and engage their team members fully.

The team will rely on their PM for direction, guidance, and support. Cultivating strong leadership skills means approaching every situation with compassion and understanding. By bringing the team members together, making them feel valued, and fostering a spirit of teamwork and cooperation, you can establish yourself as an effective leader.

Controlling

For the PM it is crucial to constantly monitor the performance of the team members during project activities. This helps to ensure that they are meeting performance metrics and standards. Periodic evaluations are also necessary to assess how well the team has achieved project goals and objectives. If monitoring and evaluations reveal that desired standards are not being met, corrective measures must be taken to improve the team's performance. This process is known as controlling.

Imagine your team is responsible for improving certain health practices of members of the project communities, such as the use of hygienic latrines that the project installs, or women giving birth at health centers instead of at their homes. If monitoring or evaluation shows that these practices are not taking place at an acceptable level, as the PM, you would need to take corrective steps. This may involve further training for team members, analyzing the situation with the contractors responsible for installing latrines, or recruiting and training more midwives for health centers. By taking timely corrective measures, you can prevent further deterioration of the project outcomes.

Successful PMs also *prioritize* and *delegate* their tasks. With many demanding tasks to complete on any given day, it is essential to prioritize tasks and delegate some to appropriate team members. This allows the PM to focus on matters of higher importance and urgency.

Project management skills and talents

The PM must possess certain essential skills to effectively manage a team. Providing clear instructions to team members regarding their tasks and arranging appropriate training are crucial steps to ensure their success. Additionally, providing necessary facilities and supplies is essential for their productivity.

However, despite best efforts, failures may occur that are beyond the PM's control. Instead of placing blame on others, a wise PM takes responsibility and strives to improve the situation while ensuring team members have what they need to carry out their tasks.

To improve one's management style, it is vital to develop necessary skills such as *decisiveness, confidence, creativity, effective communication, a positive attitude, willingness to take risks,* and *the willingness to seek increased responsibility.* Before we discuss these important skills, there is one particular skill that should be emphasized. This is the *learning* skill without which the PM will not be able to master the other skills.

Learning skill

As a global health PM, it is crucial to learn about the perspectives, priorities, and expectations of project stakeholders. An important stakeholder is the community in which the project operates. Visiting these communities and engaging in discussions with community leaders and members to gather their views, priorities, and concerns can greatly assist in project management.

Additionally, visiting hard-to-reach health centers and speaking with staff who work under difficult conditions with low resources can provide valuable insights into the needs the project aims to meet. This contributes to the PM's understanding and learning about global health issues and the project they manage.

Conversing with MOH staff at the district and sub-district levels about the project's goals and objectives can also help clarify government priorities and constraints. By observing, discussing, and interacting with stakeholders in the field, the PM can gain a better understanding of the realities on the ground. This insight is vital for effective *planning*, *organizing*, *leading*, and *controlling* the project, which are the core functions of project management.

Decisiveness

Effective managers are known for their decisiveness. The PM must clearly communicate expectations and guidelines to their team members. This will enable the team to understand what the PM requires of them. The PM's primary focus should be on achieving project results. To be results-driven, one needs to gather as much information as possible, analyze it, and consider all viable solutions. Consulting with the teammates and others outside the team can provide valuable information and insights. This helps the PM to take the best course of action when there is a decision to be made. It is crucial to do this quickly especially if the decision is time-sensitive, and you would want to do this without appearing indecisive to others.

Confidence

One can learn to become more decisive; a more effective communicator; a problem solver; a coach and mentor; and gain many other leadership skills. However, if the PM lacks personal confidence and does not believe they can lead, managing the project team can become difficult or impossible. Nobel Prize winner scientist Marie Curie once said, "*We must have perseverance and above all confidence in ourselves. We must believe that we are gifted for something, and that this thing, at whatever cost, must be attained.*"

Not only do PMs themselves need to gain self-confidence, but they also need to instill confidence among their teammates. A self-assured manager values the ideas and opinions of their team and takes pride in encouraging and empowering their teammates. Treating teammates respectfully and instilling self-confidence in them will earn you their trust and foster a healthy working environment.

Creativity

PMs demonstrate their creativity by motivating their team to generate and refine innovative ideas for implementing the health project. By doing so, the project team members will feel more satisfied with their work and be driven by their passion. To become a creative leader, it is important to study and analyze emerging data and trends and encourage the team to invent creative strategies and ideas.

Effective communication

For a manager, effective communication with their team and other stakeholders is absolutely essential. A PM needs a steady flow of accurate information for making project decisions. Therefore, all PMs must be good communicators, promoting clear and correct exchange of information. At all times the team members would need to know what the PM expects of them. And the PM would need to know what the project staff are doing. Also critical is to know what the community, donor agency, and the implementing organization's senior management expect from the project. PMs must always be aware of 'who needs what information and when,' making sure they have it.

To excel as a PM, you need to master speaking, writing, listening, and non-verbal communication. Effective communication involves understanding others, staying informed, making correct judgments, participating in meetings, and sharing information.

Teamwork hinges on successful communication among team members. To foster this in the project team, the PM needs to engage in conversations 'with' their teammates rather than talking 'at' them. During conversations, good communicators use positive body language – non-verbal gesturing – to convey their full engagement. Successful PMs actively listen when teammates speak, as listening is a crucial communication skill. Chapter 6 gives more details on the PM's communication skills.

Positive attitude

Successful PMs think positively, do positive things, and surround themselves with positive individuals. Their team members want to follow them, because of their positive attitude. Sir Winston Churchill believed, *"Attitude is a little thing that makes a big difference."*

Developing and always maintaining such a positive attitude may not be easy, especially in a high-pressured role such as the PM of a global health project. However, you can instill in yourself a positive outlook by adopting a positive perspective, becoming a more likable colleague and leader, reducing tension in your team when conflicts arise, and maintaining credibility. It may take effort, but cultivating a positive mindset is crucial to being a successful PM.

Willingness to take risks

Managing a complex health project often requires taking risks. While trying out a new strategy may not always result in the desired outcome, it is still worth pursuing. Predicting the outcome is only sometimes possible, but that should not keep the PM from taking calculated risks. Mark Zuckerberg, the co-founder of Facebook and Meta Platforms, thinks, *"The biggest risk is not taking any risk. In a world that's changing really quickly, the only strategy that is guaranteed to fail is not taking risks."*

It is prudent for the PM to consider all possible risks and prepare well to mitigate them. Effective project management involves establishing processes ahead of time to address any issues, risks, or unexpected events that may arise.

Willingness to seek increased responsibility

While some may be content with their current workload and rely on their superiors to assign them more tasks, a passionate and driven PM on the other hand, actively seeks out additional responsibilities. They constantly strive to perform at a higher level and take on challenging tasks. Exceptional PMs do not become overly concerned about taking on additional workload. To achieve success in their career, smart individuals learn to delegate some of their current responsibilities to their teammates and take on new ones.

Technical skills

The skills discussed above can be grouped into two broad categories: Conceptual skills and Human skills. Conceptual skills involve the ability to analyze a situation, identify the root cause, and understand the effect. On the other hand, human skills involve the ability to understand and influence the behaviors of individuals and groups.

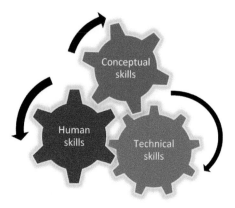

Figure 1.3 Skillset necessary for project management

In addition to these two, there is a third set of skills – *technical skills* – which are also important in project management. These pertain to job-specific knowledge and techniques needed to perform effectively in the PM role. For example, the PM who is managing a malaria control project must understand the necessary steps needed to reduce the incidence of malaria in the project area. If a project involves multiple interventions such as child nutrition, reproductive health, and HIV-TB control, a general understanding of these interventions and activities, and how they contribute to the project's goals is critical.

Your technical knowledge and skills will be rooted in your education in global health. Completing university courses in global health that especially emphasize community health will serve you well to grasp the strategies and techniques that your project will likely employ in an LMIC setting. And your practical experience in the field will further develop your technical skillset upon this academic foundation.

Your technical skills represent the 'science' of project management while your conceptual and human skills represent the 'art' of managing your project. Figure 1.3 gives a visual representation of these three skill components of project management functioning together. To excel in the role of a PM, it is critical to master and integrate both the art and the science of managing projects.

Project management styles

Throughout the years, numerous management researchers and authors have analyzed different approaches to management and leadership. They have identified various management styles in organizations, but team leaders primarily utilize four styles to lead their teams: autocratic, democratic, laissez-faire, and transformational.[4]

Autocratic style

A PM who follows an autocratic or authoritarian leadership style makes all the decisions and gives orders to the team from the top, without seeking any input or feedback from the subordinates. This kind of leader exercises absolute power and control over the team, directing them on what to do, how to do it, and where to do it. There is no dialogue or debate involved, and the team members are expected to comply with the PM's orders without question. As is the case with all the styles, the autocratic management style has its pros and cons.

Pros – In certain situations, like emergencies or chaotic environments, an authoritarian manager can be effective and make prompt decisions that the team needs to follow. In such circumstances, an autocratic approach is quite appropriate. The PM needs to make prompt decisions and the team needs to follow the decisions made. There is no room for getting everyone's input and debating the best course of action.

> I was once visiting from the U.S. headquarters of my organization a health project team in Maiduguri, Borno State of northern Nigeria when armed insurgents violently attacked the town one night. The local project team and I had made plans for training and site visits to district health centers, but the atrocities broke out when some of the planned activities were still incomplete. The PM of the local team made a quick decision to abort the rest of our planned activities and evacuate the team from that town. The PM made a swift resolve and everyone complied with the PM's decision. This was a good example of an autocratic approach to project management.

Cons – The team members working under an autocratic PM usually feel micro-managed and frustrated as they have no opportunity to contribute to any decision-making process. The team becomes overly dependent on the authoritarian manager for all directions, which can lead to a lack of creativity and motivation.

Democratic style

This approach is completely opposite to the autocratic style of project management. Also called the *participative* style of management, this approach has the PM encouraging the team members to actively engage in decision making. If you are a democratic manager, you value the ideas and opinions of your team and solicit their input in planning and problem-solving. While ultimately responsible for making the final decision, you empower your team to have a say in the process.

As a democratic team leader, the PM prioritizes getting input from everyone on their team and is known for their effective communication skills and approachability. They are open to ideas and feedback, even if these differ from their own. Democratic PMs take responsibility for their team's failures and recognize the contributions of team members toward project success.

Pros – When each team member contributes to the decision-making process, the PM can make informed decisions with multiple inputs that lead to the desired results. This fosters a sense of mutual respect among team members, ultimately boosting team morale. This democratic or participative approach has been proven to produce higher quality performance and job satisfaction, making it widely recognized as a very effective management method.

Cons – It is important to recognize the skillset of the team and not overestimate their abilities in areas they may not be trained in. Expecting too much can lead to disappointment and unproductive outcomes. Additionally, considering everyone's input can delay progress as group decision-making can take time, which may hinder the attainment of project targets.

Laissez-faire style

This leadership style, also known as the *delegative* approach, grants team members the autonomy to run project activities with minimal direction from the team leader. A laissez-faire PM entrusts the team with the power to complete their tasks without micro-management. The PM's role is to offer feedback when needed while leaving decision-making in the hands of the team members.

Pros – In circumstances where team members possess adequate experience and confidence in completing project tasks and making decisions on their own, adopting a 'hands off' approach can prove to be highly effective. This can expedite the decision-making process, as subordinates do not need to seek approval from their manager for everything. By functioning independently and employing creative methods, team members feel a greater sense of accomplishment and confidence when empowered to execute their work without constant interference or direction from the PM.

Cons – If the project team members lack a clear understanding of their tasks, or if there is lack of experience or confidence within the team, adopting a laissez-faire approach can have disastrous consequences. Without proper guidance and oversight, the team may fail to accomplish anything, and it may be necessary for the PM to abandon this delegative style of management.

Transformational style

A PM who adopts a transformational approach develops a compelling vision for the project and motivates team members to work towards it. Working under such a leader, team members are united in achieving the project goal and are willing to dedicate their time and energy to attain it. This leadership style transforms team members both personally and professionally, making them enthusiastic about working together to realize the project's objectives and targets.

Pros – The transformational management approach is beneficial in enabling team members to fully understand and appreciate the ambitious goals set by their PM. This helps to foster loyalty towards the leader while increasing productivity towards the project objectives. A harmonious environment is established within the team, where communication between team members and their leader remains open and honest.

Cons – When the transformational PM sets ambitious goals for their team, there is a risk of burnout. To prevent this, it is crucial for the PM to maintain constant communication with their team. If communication breaks down for any reason, the team may feel ignored, disconnected, and discouraged.

A practical management style

After considering the four principal management styles, you may be wondering which one would suit you best. Unfortunately, there is no easy answer to this question. Each approach has its advantages and disadvantages, as discussed above. It would be ideal to utilize all four styles in managing your project team, incorporating various aspects from each style as necessary.[5]

When working on a project, it may be necessary to enforce strict guidelines due to organizational, government, or donor agency regulations. For example, if the donor agency requires quotes from three contractors for building a pharmaceutical warehouse or printing health educational materials, the PM may need to take an autocratic management approach to ensure strict compliance from team members who are unfamiliar with the regulation.

In situations where there are no strict guidelines, a democratic management style may be preferred. This approach allows for maximum input from the team when making decisions and solving problems.

There may be instances where utilizing the laissez-faire management style could be appropriate. For instance, if the project team is highly skilled and enthusiastic about conducting routine training sessions for government health center midwives on performing normal deliveries and managing post-partum hemorrhage, there may not be a need for an autocratic or democratic leader. Adopting a laissez-faire approach to team management in this situation could be beneficial, as the PM is confident in the team's abilities and potentials.

If a PM has an ambitious goal for their project, considering the use of the transformational management style with the existing team can be advantageous. For example, if the PM wants to expand the malaria control project to three new districts within a year, this will require extra effort. By using the transformational style, the PM can motivate their team members to support this vision and work together to accomplish it successfully.

To be an effective PM, one needs to be adaptable and flexible in their project management strategy. This means being able to choose the appropriate approach for each unique situation and skillfully combining or sequencing different styles as needed. Experts in leadership consider this *practical* style to be the most successful approach to managing a project team.

Project completion

The last phase of the global health project life is its completion phase. The project has delivered what it promised, and the stakeholders are satisfied with the results. It is now time to draw the project to a close. There are specific tasks that the PM must carry out to ensure this phase is done correctly.

Undertaking end-of-project evaluation

With the assistance of the MEAL team, the PM is responsible for conducting a final evaluation of the project, also known as the end-of-project evaluation. The report produced from this evaluation primarily focuses on the project's accomplishments, its impact on community members and partners, any obstacles encountered, lessons learned, and recommendations for stakeholders. It is essential to disseminate the final evaluation report to all parties involved in the project's implementation, including community leaders and members, the donor agency, MOH officials, and senior staff of the implementing organization. See Chapter 10.

Sending official letters and organizing closure meetings

The PM formally notifies the important stakeholders through letters and official meetings regarding the successful completion of the project.

Holding a project closure meeting with the communities where the project was implemented is crucial, and yet often neglected. Sharing project accomplishments and the valuable insights gained from the final evaluation with community leaders and members brings a sense of closure to their connection with the project team. Marking the project's success with the community is a great way to conclude the project.

Closing project contract

Some projects are performed under contracts with the funding agency or with the MOH and others. The PM is responsible for properly documenting and finalizing all project records. This includes capturing, among other things, the final results of the project, which can be the final evaluation report. To ensure all reports, including financial reports, are completed, and submitted correctly, it is important to consult with the implementing organization's headquarters staff that oversee project contracts. If certifications on the project performance are needed from external agencies, the PM obtains them for the records.

Celebrating the project accomplishments

It is important for the project team to acknowledge their achievements and for the PM to formally appreciate their contributions, thank them for their involvement, and officially wrap up the project. Celebrating the success of the project helps team members to acknowledge its completion and brings a sense of closure to the hard work they put in. It also inspires them to reflect on their learnings and consider how their experiences can benefit both themselves and their organization in future projects.

Recognizing progress and celebrating small victories along the way is equally important as doing these at the project's closing. Nelson Mandela said, "*Remember to celebrate milestones as you prepare for the road ahead.*"

The inspiring PM encourages their teammates throughout the project duration by acknowledging and celebrating their accomplishments at every turn in the path, even while planning for the journey ahead.

Difficulties in health project management

As we conclude this chapter, it is important to point out some practical challenges PMs often face. Be aware of these potential issues, remain watchful, and do not allow these problems to bring you down. Being a

PM, particularly someone who is a novice, can be a complex, stressful, and frustrating experience at times. There are a few reasons for this, such as:

Lack of training on new responsibilities, leadership techniques, and methods of managing people. PMs may have excelled in a *technical* role but are now faced with new and diverse challenges in a *management* role.

The intimidation of enforcing various policies and procedures, some of which may be technical or legal in nature. The PMs must be accountable for all of them, even if they do not fully understand them.

Limited time to monitor department progress and maintain relationships with a diverse range of people from different backgrounds even while managing and guiding them.

High stress levels, which can be daunting to admit, particularly to their superiors who already have high expectations of the PM.

The feeling of isolation in their PM role, especially if they were promoted over their former colleagues. They must meet the needs of their superiors while also ensuring their subordinates are looked after.

There is no secret formula to overcoming these challenges, but the more prepared you are for assuming the role of PM, the easier it becomes. The following chapters aim to help you prepare for that role.

"Success is no accident. It is hard work, perseverance, learning, studying, sacrifice and most of all, the love of what you are doing or learning to do." – Pele.

Key takeaways

- Organizations such as the MOH or NGOs implement health projects to improve the health of a population.
- Main features of health projects are its input, process, output, and outcome.
- Success is measured not only by meeting goals but also by fulfilling stakeholder expectations.
- A global health project goes through four basic phases: *the planning phase, the implementing phase, the Monitoring phase, and the Evaluating phase.* These may overlap with one another.
- Health projects are operated by teams of trained individuals who share common health goals and objectives.

- Global health projects have different types of interventions and, therefore, are run by different types of project teams.
- The PM ensures the team composition and training match the types of project interventions.
- As the PM, you will need to plan, organize, lead, and control your team and other resources for achieving project goals, objectives, and outcomes. In addition to these four central functions, you ought to prioritize and delegate tasks to team members.
- The PM must also have a clear vision for their project and its success.
- For the day-to-day operation of their project, PMs need to do micro-planning, which is the DAP.
- Decisiveness, confidence, creativity, effective communication, a positive attitude, willingness to take risks, and the willingness to seek increased responsibility are the hallmark skills that can help the PM manage their project.
- There are many styles to utilize in managing a project. The four basic ones are the *autocratic, democratic, laissez-faire, and transformational styles.* Ideally, you would utilize all four styles as necessary in different circumstances.
- It is important to celebrate project accomplishments so that team members gain a sense of closure to their work as well as inspiration for utilizing their learnings and experiences in future projects.
- If you are the PM of a project, especially if you are a new PM, you may at times experience confusion, frustration, and stress in your role. In the words of Pele: "*Success is no accident. It is hard work, perseverance, learning, studying, sacrifice and most of all, the love of what you are doing or learning to do.*"

Discussion questions

1. A global health project can achieve its goals and objectives but still not be considered a successful project. Do you agree with this statement? Why or why not?
2. How will you ensure your team is meeting performance metrics and standards during project operation?
3. What is meant by the 'art' and the 'science' of project management?
4. Why is it important to celebrate your project accomplishments?
5. Table 1.1 contains five numbered items covered in this chapter, with short descriptions in the right column. However, these descriptions are not arranged in the correct order and do not match the items on the left. Match each numbered item to its description on the right and correctly write the corresponding letter of the description in the middle column.

Table 1.1 Multiple choice questions

Match the following with the answers in the last column	Insert letter of the correct answer	Answer
1. NGO run projects		A. The changes in the community that the project brings about.
2. Examples of project inputs are		B. Plan, organize, lead, and control the human and other resources available
3. Project outcomes are		C. Assist the government (MOH) to provide healthcare to the communities.
4. Basic role of the PMs is to		D. Team members share their ideas and views.
5. Under the democratic style of project management		E. Project staff, funding, vehicles, office space, etc.

See correct answers on page 194.

Case study exercise

As the newly appointed PM of a child nutrition project in an LMIC, you are managing a team with varying levels of experience. While some team members are confident in their responsibilities, there are others that are new to the project and are still adjusting. The project (1) provides health education to village mothers on feeding nutritious food to their children; (2) distributes nutrition supplements to government health centers, and (3) refers severely malnourished children to medical facilities for nutrition intervention. There are other activities, but these are the most important ones.

Your team members responsible for giving health education are performing well. However, there are issues with referring severely malnourished children to the appropriate facilities and there are delays in distributing nutrition supplements from the project stock to the health centers.

What management style will you employ in making sure that your team is functioning at an optimum level, and what steps will you take to ensure all project activities are accomplished?

See Author's suggestion on page 195.

Notes

1 Rosemary McMahon, Elizabeth Barton & Maurice Piot, *On Being in Charge: A Guide to Management in Primary Health Care* (Geneva: World Health Organization, 1992), 47.
2 Gareth R. Jones and Jennifer M. George, *Essentials of Contemporary Management* (New York: McGraw-Hill/Irwin, 2009), 5.

3 "What is 'Management'? What Do Managers Do?" *Management Library,* last modified May 18, 2023, accessed June 23, 2023, https://management. org/management/guidebook.htm#anchor1012225
4 "4 Leadership Styles in Business: Leadership Style Quiz," last updated June 17, 2022, accessed April 19, 2023, www.uagc.edu/blog/4-leadership-styles-in-business.
5 Chelsea Levinson, "Different Supervisory Styles of Managers," *Bizfluent, last modified January 28, 2022,* https://bizfluent.com/info-7736754-different-supervisory-styles-managers.html. 28 January 2022.

References

"4 Leadership Styles in Business: Leadership Style Quiz." *The University of Arizona Global Campus.* Last updated June 17, 2022. www.uagc.edu/blog/4-leadership-styles-in-business

Jones, Gareth R. and Jennifer M. George. 2009. *Essentials of Contemporary Management* (New York: McGraw-Hill/Irwin.

Levinson, Chelsea. 2022. "Different Supervisory Styles of Managers." *Bizfluent.* Last modified January 28. https://bizfluent.com/info-7736754-different-supervisory-styles-managers.html. 28 January 2022.

Management Library. 2023. "What is 'Management'? What Do Managers Do?" Last modified May 18. https://management.org/management/guidebook. htm#anchor1012225

McMahon, Rosemary and Elizabeth Barton & Maurice Piot. 1992. *On Being in Charge: A Guide to Management in Primary Health Care.* Geneva: World Health Organization.

2 Building global health project teams

Global health and global health project team

In the previous chapter, you learned some of the fundamental aspects of global health project. The remaining chapters of this book provide in-depth insights on how to manage critical aspects of such projects. These include developing project activity plans, enhancing project team performance, monitoring and evaluating project activities and outcomes, tracking budgets, and more. However, none of these can be accomplished unless the PM, as the leader, establishes a strong and motivated team of trained individuals. Operating a global health project is not a one-person job. It takes a team of qualified individuals. To take a piece of advice from the business world, *"Great things in business are never done by one person. They're done by a team of people."* – Steve Jobs, co-founder, former chairman, and CEO of Apple.

Successful projects need effective teams with robust and trusting relationships between the PM and their team members and between themselves. They also need a clear vision and objectives, adequate resources, guidelines, and constant team communications. They should also be empowered to make collective decisions and solve work-related problems.

This chapter is written early on in the book to show you how the selection of team members take place, how the PM guides the interactions and support for project teams, and how they ensure the teams understand the health project, and individual roles and responsibilities. First though we need to define global health and project teams.

Different health organizations and institutions have varying emphases when they define global health and global health teams. Some focus on the 'global' aspect while others prioritize 'equitable access' to healthcare. At Duke University's Global Health Institute, global health is defined as 'strategies that achieve better health outcomes for vulnerable populations and communities around the world.' It emphasizes a broad, multidisciplinary approach to understanding emerging health challenges, considering social, cultural, economic, and environmental factors that underlie health inequities.[1] This is the definition we will use in this book for global health.

DOI: 10.4324/9781003405245-3

A global health project team consists of trained staff who work together to achieve common goals and respond to the health needs of the community they serve. Support staff, such as those in human resources (HR), logistics, and finance departments, as well as drivers and cleaners, provide assistance to multiple projects (health and non-health) in the same country and may be based in the same country office. In most cases they are 'shared staff' and not normally considered members of the global health project team as they do not always report to the PM. They generally report to their own departmental heads. However, there are instances where the support staff are part of the project team and managed by the PM or other senior team members.

Health projects and project teams are of diverse types, depending on the nature of their work. Some are mobile or ambulatory teams traveling to various places to provide health care services to far-flung communities. As an example, during the 2014–2016 West Africa Ebola Virus Disease outbreak, both government and non-government organizations launched mobile teams in Guinea, Liberia, and Sierra Leone to provide prevention and treatment services.

On the other hand, stationary teams are based in one location and work in a single office. While they may still need to travel to and from local project sites, their main office serves as the central hub for communication and coordination. Vehicles and other team assets are kept at this central location. Such a base office, also called a national office or country office, may have its location in the capital of a country or a large city nearby. It is usual for a project to also have satellite offices on project *sites*. Some team members are stationed in these site offices reporting to their immediate supervisors at the project site, or to more senior supervisors in the national or country office. These sites also have vehicles, office space, and other assets just like that of the central office, only in a smaller scale. Image 2.1 shows a local health project team gathered for a meeting at a project site.

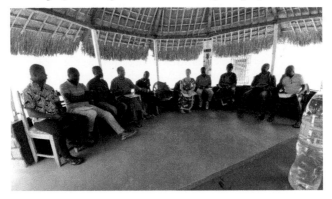

Image 2.1 Team meeting at a remote project site in Central African Republic

The PM of a global health project in an LMIC is responsible for leading and coordinating the entire team, regardless of their location. It is the PM's duty to ensure that all team members (at site offices and at the base office) work together towards achieving the project's objectives and goals. To accomplish this, the PM needs a team with diverse skills and roles. Some team members may specialize in staff training, who trains other staff in various areas, health educators to educate communities on health matters, or individuals that supervise peripheral staff. Depending on the type of project and the type of organization running it, team structures and composition may vary. Nonetheless, a simple team structure commonly used by many organizations is discussed in the next section.

Key positions in a health project team

In this section, we will outline the structure of an illustrative project team responsible for preventing and treating TB in an LMIC. In this model an international NGO conceived of this project and secured funding from donor agencies. The project aims to collaborate with the MOH of the country, including its district and sub-district government health offices. The collaboration takes place through the project team. The project goal is to contribute to the MOH objective of decreasing the TB burden in the country.

The PM of the TB project (sometimes also referred to as 'Chief of Party') heads the team with the overall responsibility for the success of the project. Depending on the project's size, there may be one or more assistant project managers (APMs) who report to the PM and oversee project officers (POs) and training coordinators (TCs).

An APM might supervise several POs, one or more TCs, as well as support staff, such as the finance and human resource personnel, project drivers, office maintenance staff, and other non-technical staff if they are included in the project team.

The POs supervise more peripheral level team members, such as community health promoters (CHPs), who in turn supervise the CHWs and community health volunteers (CHVs). Figure 2.1 depicts a simple health project team staffing structure (organogram) with five levels.

The team's staffing structure may vary depending on the project's needs and design. For instance, the team may include a laboratory technician (LT) who supports the government laboratory facilities in detecting TB, or a monitoring and evaluation (MEAL) specialist who monitors the project's progress and evaluates its effectiveness. These staff members included in the project team report to the PM or an APM.

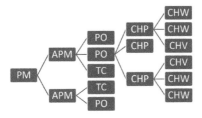

Figure 2.1 A simplified organogram of a health project team

It is worth noting that the job titles of team members may differ from country to country. For example, a 'CHW' in one country may be called a 'health agent' in another country, or an 'Anganwadi worker' in yet another place. However, the functions of each category of team members in most global health projects are quite similar.

In some cases, an NGO may have multiple projects, both health and non-health, operating simultaneously in the same region or district of the same LMIC. In such cases, support staff work across different projects without belonging to any specific project team. There are exceptions, however, as mentioned above. These support staff schedule and budget their time across the projects that use their services when not part of a single project. All these projects operating in that country benefit from their services. Thus, multiple projects cover their remunerations, benefits, and travel costs, etc., with their individual project budgets.

It is generally recommended that individuals in supervisory roles, such as PMs, APMs, POs, and CHPs, oversee no more than 15 employees. When a supervisor manages too many individuals, the task of supervision can become overwhelming. Typically, successful projects have one supervisor for every 5 to 10 employees. The PM and other centrally placed staff usually have fewer employees to supervise relative to the other supervisors in the team as they have additional managerial responsibilities. On the other hand, peripherally placed staff in supervisory roles may have a larger number of individuals to oversee.

Developing job aids and job descriptions

Following graduation you may be recruited to manage a global health project in an LMIC. You may encounter one of two situations. In the first scenario, you are the PM leading a team that is already established, with most of the key positions filled. You have an APM, a number of POs, CHPs, and other categories of staff in your team. This means you will need to work with and lead an existing team. Let us name this scenario 'S1' for convenience of discussion.

In the second scenario, which we will call 'S2,' imagine your organization has appointed you as the PM for a *new* project where the team has not yet been formed. Your responsibilities will include recruiting staff and leading them, although there may not be much information available about the specific job description of their positions. However, you do have support staff in your country office, or your implementing organization's headquarters or regional office who can assist you with staff recruitment, onboarding, and placement.

In both S1 and S2 scenarios, the PM will need to hire new staff members for building up the health project team. This need is more urgent in S2, but turnover, resignations, contract terminations, and retirements may also occur time to time in the S1 scenario. Thus, staff recruitment also takes place in S1. Additionally, new positions may need to be created and staffed to meet project demands or address gaps in performance in either scenario. As the PM, it is your responsibility to fill any staff vacancies promptly and thoughtfully in S1 and S2.

The PM creates job aids and job descriptions to assist their teams in performing their tasks accurately and improving their work. It is essential to determine if job descriptions or job aids for team positions already exist. If not, the HR department can assist in creating these vital tools, which are necessary for recruiting team members and helping them to perform their tasks well.

When reviewing job descriptions and job aids or creating new ones it is important to align them with the project's requirements. The PM is the best person to determine the roles and responsibilities of each position. Therefore, they request the HR department to create an official job description. For instance, if a trained pharmacist is needed to assist government pharmacists in the MOH health centers with ordering and storing medicines, a job description must be developed (if not already available) to recruit and then guide a qualified pharmacist. Additionally, if a job description needs to include an extra task, the PM notifies the HR department so they can update an existing job description. Job aids and job descriptions show team members how to effectively perform their tasks and allow their PM to evaluate their performance.

Job aids

Job aids are clear and concise written guides that assist project staff in completing their tasks quickly and accurately. By using job aids, team members can reduce the number of errors they might make and complete their work procedures much more efficiently. Job aids can have various formats, with a simple and practical option being a step-by-step listing of tasks and sub-tasks. The addition of pictures and infographics enhances the clarity and engagement of the job aid. Video tutorials are also useful online formats for job aids.

A job aid provides easy-to-follow instructions for project staff, such as the steps to take for detecting severely malnourished children using the mid-upper arm circumference (MUAC) tape and referring them to the proper treatment facility, or things to do for educating caregivers on how to prepare ORS solution at home for sick children.

To create a job aid, the PM or someone familiar with the project tasks can follow these steps.

Step 1. Identifying who will use the job aid

When creating a job aid, one needs to identify its intended user and purpose. The PM considers the advantages it will provide, and which members of the team will benefit from it. They determine the critical stage in the teammate's workflow where they might need to use the job aid.

Step 2. Collecting task related information

The PM lists all the steps the user of the job aid needs to follow to get the task done successfully. Including reminders and precautions, tips, or alternative ways to complete the task and sub-tasks is helpful. A list of frequently asked questions and common mistakes related to the particular task is beneficial to include in the job aid.

Step 3. Creating a draft job aid

To create a set of clear instructions, the PM chooses a format such as step-by-step sequential listing of tasks and sub-tasks that the user of the job aid will follow. For example, if the need is to instruct a team member who monitors vaccines in a cold chain facility, the PM should create a job aid that explains how the individual will read the thermometer on the refrigerator, how the temperature will be recorded using a logbook or chart, how often one should record it, and how to activate a backup system during a power outage. By listing these tasks and sub-tasks in an organized manner, the PM makes it easier for the job aid user to recall the essential functions required to monitor the cold chain facility.

Step 4. Testing and finalizing the job aid

The next stage in creating a job aid is to undertake a field test and finalize it. To continue with the example above, the PM puts to test the draft job aid during an actual visit to a cold chain facility.

The PM will need to use it with their team member (the vaccine monitor) who monitors cold chain facilities to determine if the individual can understand the draft job aid and perform in a logical manner all the tasks and sub-tasks listed in it. Together, they assess if the job aid is easily understandable and if it enables the user to complete all the tasks and sub-tasks in a logical sequence. For example, the job aid may instruct the user to "Read the temperature from the thermometer on the refrigerator" and "Record the temperature with time and date of inspection in the appropriate space on the facility chart." The PM observes as the vaccine monitor uses the job aid to determine if the tool is effective in explaining the tasks, or if changes are necessary. Based on this field testing necessary revisions and adjustments are made before finalizing the job aid. Once the job aid is finalized, the PM provides clear instructions to the team member on how to use it. The PM may decide to delegate to a senior supervisor (e.g., APM or PO) this task of testing the tool at the cold chain facility with the job aid user.

Job descriptions

While job aids give instructions on how a staff will complete specific tasks and sub-tasks, job descriptions on the other hand clarify the *role* of each team member working on the health project. All team members need to have specific job descriptions that guide their roles and functions.

Each job description should begin with the position title (e.g., project officer) and summarize the overall role of a particular position. The job description should then include a list of the specific tasks the individual in that position will perform. Some examples from such a list can be:

"Visit X number of project sites each month to monitor health center construction work. Use the monitoring checklist to identify completion or gaps in the construction activities;" (appropriate for a project site manager or a monitoring officer). Note, unlike a job aid the job description does not tell the staff the detailed steps of how to monitor the construction work; nor how or where to record the findings from the monitoring visit.

"Organize one health education session on child nutrition each week for community mothers in X number of project sites" (applicable for a CHW).

"Train X number of CHWs on malaria prevention strategies each month using visuals, such as flip books; and engaging participants to do a skit or drama that is related to the specific session topic" (ideal for a TC, CHP, or a PO).

There is usually other information in a formal job description. It specifies where the position is based (e.g., Country Office/City, or project site and district). It mentions the position to whom this person is reportable, (e.g., Reportable to APM). If the position is a supervisory one, the job description specifies who and how many staff the individual is to supervise (e.g., "The PO will supervise six to eight CHPs").

Selecting team members

Now that the PM has the job description and the job aid prepared, selecting the right candidates to join their team becomes simplified. The HR Department is responsible for posting job vacancies and screening applicants. They create the vacancy announcement based on the job description and job aid. In the announcement the department with inputs from the PM and their team outlines the job functions, minimum education, and professional requirements that the applicants must meet.

Appendix-A gives a sample job description for an APM. A fictitious organization, XYZ Agency is using this illustrative job description to make a vacancy announcement for recruiting an APM in Ukraine for a global health and nutrition project.

HR reviews the applications which it receives in response to the vacancy announcement, and then shortlists potential candidates for interviews. The PM and senior team members use the shortlist to conduct interviews and select the best candidate. The HR negotiates with the top candidate, performs background checks, and extends a job offer to the selected individual. The HR Department also assists with the signing of employment agreements, onboarding, orientation, and all official steps that are necessary for the candidate to start functioning in the team. Once onboard the PM and other team members provide orientation on project related areas, and the new hire then begins working as part of the team.

It is advisable for the PM to work closely with HR during the candidate selection process. The notes shared by HR from candidate screening or reviewing their Curriculum Vitae (CV) should be taken into consideration. It can be tempting to overlook the advice or red flags raised by HR about certain candidates. However, in spite of the fact that they are not necessarily health professionals, colleagues in the HR department can offer a generalist's perspective that technically oriented individuals often miss.

It is possible that there could be obvious or subtle pressure to hire a specific candidate. However, a competent PM will stand firm and overcome any such pressure, only selecting the most suitable candidates for the job. The chosen individuals should be capable of fulfilling the requirements outlined in their job description.

It is not uncommon for some to justify hiring a less qualified candidate with the belief that they can be trained and brought up to speed to meet the expected work standards. While training and mentoring can certainly improve the performance of newly recruited individuals, it should never come at the cost of compromising the basic minimum requirements listed in the job description and vacancy announcement. For example, if the position requires a nurse with three years of experience, it would be unwise to hire someone with only one year of experience just because they are fluent in the local language. Project training cannot replace the necessary nursing experience required for the position. Similarly, hiring someone who is still a final-year college student, despite the minimum requirement being a college graduate with a degree, should not be acceptable. It is imperative that the basic minimum requirements are met for every individual hired to ensure the formation of a strong project team.

If for valid reasons (such as no candidate is available that meets the minimum requirements) recruitment is stalled, then the PM should carefully review and revise the job description, particularly the minimum requirements. However, it is important for the PM to avoid the temptation or pressure of altering these requirements solely to accommodate a preferred candidate.

To make progress in the health project, the PM needs a team that is willing to accept their leadership and work together. Cooperation from everyone involved, including stakeholders outside of the team, is essential. However, it is not beneficial for the PM to only hire people who agree with them. Surrounding oneself with 'Yes-Men' is not the best approach. Instead, experienced PMs seek out individuals who can bring creative solutions to the table, even if they sometimes disagree with them. This will lead to better planning, project execution, and problem-solving.

It is important to motivate every member of the team to participate actively in the planning, problem-solving, innovation, and development of the project. To achieve the best results, the PM needs to create an environment where everyone – particularly the newly recruited teammates – feels comfortable expressing their thoughts and ideas, and where their contributions are valued and taken into consideration.

Directing project teams

Once a health project team has been formed, it requires consistent direction, guidance, support, and feedback from its team leader. The PM's leading the team can vary from direct involvement in ongoing tasks to a more supportive role. The various types of management styles have been discussed in details in Chapter 1.

To effectively lead the health project team, the PM must focus on several critical areas that are applicable to all PM roles. These areas of leadership typically involve *visioning, motivating, delegating*, and *supervising*. Although there are other important aspects of leadership, we will only discuss these key areas in this chapter, except for the topic of team 'supervision,' which requires a separate and more in-depth discussion, as done in Chapter 5.

Developing and sharing project vision

To successfully guide project teams PMs must have a well-defined vision of the desired outcomes for their projects. Moreover, they must be able to clearly communicate this vision to their team members and assist them in attaining it. Industrialist and philanthropist Andrew Carnegie said, *"Teamwork is the ability to work together toward a common vision, the ability to direct individual accomplishments toward organizational objectives. It is the fuel that allows common people to attain uncommon results."* Successful PMs leverage their position, personality, persuasive abilities, power, and communication skills to influence their team members to perform at a high level and achieve their vision for the health project. This will ultimately cultivate a highly committed and motivated team,[2] with each team member fully embracing their individual roles.

Setting project objectives jointly with team members

When taking on the role of PM, one typically finds the project objectives are already established during the proposal development phase and outlined in agreements with funding agencies and/or the MOH. There can be little opportunity to freshly develop or revise these project objectives.

However, there may be instances where new objectives need to be created, such as when designing a new project or extending an existing one. After evaluations of an existing project, adjustments to its objectives, interventions, activities, and sub-activities may be necessary, and new indicators and targets may need to be developed or revisited.

In these situations, it is productive to involve team members in the process of developing these components collaboratively, whenever possible. They are more enthusiastic to achieve objectives and targets that they have helped select as opposed to those that others have set for the team.

Motivating team members

It is vital for the PM to ensure that their team members feel satisfied by utilizing their talents and skills to reach their goals. By providing them with opportunities to experience fulfillment in their work, the PM can motivate them to do what is needed for the success of the health project. Some motivating factors for team members include feeling a sense of accomplishment, receiving recognition for their contributions, comprehending the significance of their work, discovering opportunities for personal growth, and advancing their careers. When motivating team members, the PM should understand what motivates each individual.

Most individuals strive to perform well and succeed in their work. The PM can help their team members achieve a sense of success and accomplishment by providing them with clear guidance, sufficient training, and the necessary resources to perform their jobs effectively. A competent PM will do their utmost to ensure their teammates have everything they need to achieve their targets and objectives.

Success needs to be recognized. It is important to acknowledge and celebrate the success of each individual in your team. The team members take pride in their work, and by recognizing their achievements publicly the PM can create healthy competition and motivate team members to perform better. The PM assures their project teammates that their work is worthwhile and valuable in improving the health of the community where they operate their health project. When team members understand the importance of their work, they are more likely to give their best effort.

To help team members grow and develop, far-sighted PMs offer them opportunities for personal and professional development. This can include challenging assignments, research projects, and problem-solving tasks, as well as identifying training opportunities to increase motivation. By investing in their team members, PMs can create a positive work environment that fosters success and personal growth.

Encouraging the teammates to enhance their knowledge and skills in preparation for promotion is a great way to motivate them for improved performance. Once they are ready, the PM can consider providing them with tangible recognition, such as higher responsibilities, a salary increase, or a bonus. Such career advancement opportunities can boost their job satisfaction and inspire them to work harder.

Ultimately, true long-term motivation is intrinsic, and it stems from self-motivation. Your teammates will *want* to do what you envision for your project. In the words of the 34th U.S. President Dwight Eisenhower, "*Motivation is the art of getting people to do what you want them to do because they want to do it.*" By following the suggestions outlined above, one can assist team members in fostering this type of lasting motivation for their work.

Delegating responsibilities

To build up team capabilities, it may be necessary to delegate to project team members some of the responsibilities that PMs normally undertake. Delegation involves selectively granting authority and responsibilities to a team member to execute well-defined tasks that the PM is unable to undertake due to time constraints or the need to focus on other important and urgent matters.

Delegating is an essential skill for team leaders. It requires working with team members to establish goals and targets, and giving them the authority and responsibility to achieve them. The PM must grant their delegate sufficient freedom to decide how to achieve these goals, be available as a resource to support them, evaluate their work, and reward achievements while addressing performance issues.

To give an example, the PM attends monthly meetings with external stakeholders, such as the MOH health officer at a certain district. However, if a pressing need arises, the PM may delegate this task to someone in the project team with proven qualities, such as an assistant, the APM. Delegating responsibilities saves time for other critical activities.

The delegated staff does not have to wait for the PM's approval to perform the task that the PM has already delegated, so there is no delay in executing it. Delegation allows for increasing the knowledge, skills, and motivation of the team members. It also can lead to promotion and career advancement of individuals that prove themselves with additional responsibilities. This contributes to the building of the project team.

When delegating, it is essential to consider who in the team is ready to handle the responsibilities. The team member must have the necessary skills to undertake the task and understand it well. Before delegating, it is necessary to prepare the person through coaching and mentoring so the delegate has a good understanding of the task that needs to be accomplished.

When delegating a task, it is crucial to inform all those concerned both inside and outside the project team about your decision to delegate, removing confusion and securing cooperation. After delegating a task the PM should not interfere but offer support if needed. However, following up to see how the individual has made progress with the delegated task is necessary.

One must guard against over-delegation, as the selected person must not get overwhelmed with the responsibilities the PM delegates. The PM must avoid delegating too many tasks to multiple members of their team to lessen their own workload. It is the PM who is ultimately accountable for all project work. Not the team members.

Resolving conflict

At times conflicts may arise among team members. They spend quite a bit of their time together especially when working on a complex health project that requires a lot of collaboration. These conflicts can stem from differences in opinions or difficulties in personal relationships. Cultural differences and rivalry may contribute to conflicts. It is important to address these conflicts as soon as possible to prevent harm to the project. The PM must not let bitterness fester but resolve the disputes quickly. A harmonious and unified team is crucial for achieving project goals and objectives.

As a skilled mediator, the PM's role is to resolve disputes between individuals or groups by negotiating a fair agreement. To effectively mediate a conflict, it is crucial for the PM to establish themselves as a neutral third party whose sole focus is to reach a resolution.[3] The success as a PM in this role depends on both parties perceiving them as unbiased and genuinely committed to finding a fair and just outcome.

To resolve conflicts among members of their project team, experienced PMs follow these specific steps. The PMs:

- Gather information from all parties involved and clarify the source of the conflict.
- Meet at a private and safe place to discuss the issue with all parties concerned.
- Listen with a positive and assertive approach to allow everyone to voice their opinion.
- Investigate deeper and discuss their findings separately with each party without taking sides or making a final judgment.
- Develop a common goal and articulate it to both parties. The parties discuss different options for working together towards achieving the common goal. The PMs let all parties propose options and points out their strengths and weaknesses. They encourage everyone from both sides to make some compromises.
- Help everyone agree on the best solution and specify the responsibilities of each party to work towards the resolution.
- Stay engaged to evaluate progress and ensure both parties are fulfilling their responsibilities.
- Finally, develop strategies to prevent similar conflicts in the future.

Putting yourself in the shoes of a PM, what about a situation where *you* may find yourself in conflict with one or more of your teammates?

In such situations it is important to address the issue in a way that does not hinder the progress of the project. The steps just mentioned can be applied in this scenario as well.

- It is essential to have a private conversation with the person(s) and avoid focusing on personalities.
- Instead, point out the specific behaviors and events that led to the conflict.
- Listen attentively and ask questions to gain a better understanding of their perspective. Demonstrate that you are genuinely interested in resolving the conflict.
- Together, identify the crucial areas of conflict and create a plan to resolve them.
- Set up future discussions to assess progress and follow through on the plan.
- Evaluate the outcome and recognize the efforts made by your teammate(s), genuinely complimenting the other person(s) for the progress made.[4]

As you can see, there are many areas where a PM needs to focus as they build their global health project team. But do not lose sight of the most important things that you can give to your team. In the words of Anne Sweeny, an American businesswoman and former chair and president at The Walt Disney Company, "*The greatest gift you can give your team: clarity, communication, and pulling people together around a shared mission.*"

Key takeaways

- None of the project activities can happen unless the PM carefully builds up the project team.
- A global health project team is made up of individuals working with a shared goal and objectives to respond to the health needs of the community they serve.
- The PM of a global health project team is ultimately responsible for project success. Others in the team help the PM achieve this success.
- Visioning means the PM develops a clear idea of the end result of the project and articulates this vision to the team members.
- A supervisor normally should have no more than 15 staff members to supervise. Ideally, this number should be between five and ten.
- The PM and HR use job descriptions to select and recruit project staff.
- Job aids are clear and concise written guidelines that spell out the manner in which a member of the project team is to complete a specific task.
- A job description explains the role of the team member.

- An experienced PM resists and overcomes pressures and prejudices when hiring team members. The minimum requirements for a position as specified in the vacancy announcement should be strictly followed in selecting candidates for team positions.
- Selecting those that may not always agree with you but will bring their creative alternative options to project planning, problem-solving, and project execution is a sensible strategy.
- Directing project teams entails visioning, motivating, delegating, and supervising.
- Conflict among team members and sometimes between the PM and a team member is not uncommon. It is essential to mediate between the feuding parties and find a negotiated resolution urgently.
- Conflicting parties expect the PM to play an honestly neutral and unbiased mediating role.

Discussion questions

1. What steps will you take to develop a practical job aid for a team member?
2. Before a team can achieve project activities there is a fundamental need for resolving any conflict within the project team. Do you agree with this statement? Why or why not?
3. Table 2.1 contains five numbered items covered in this chapter, with short descriptions in the right column. However, these descriptions are not arranged in the correct order and do not match the items on the left. Match each numbered item to its description on the right and correctly write the corresponding letter of the description in the middle column.

Table 2.1 Multiple choice questions

Match the following with the answers in the last column	Insert letter of the correct answer	Answer
1. Job description		A. Staff uses this to complete specific tasks
2. Job aid		B. Requires a truly neutral and unbiased mediator
3. Conflict resolution		C. Allows time for completing other activities
4. Visioning entails		D. Describes roles and responsibilities of staff
5. Delegating a task		E. Developing a clear idea of the end result

See correct answers on page 194.

Case study exercise

As the new PM of a health project in an LMIC, you have inherited a demoralized and unproductive team. Several team members hold a negative view of the previous PM, and they are unsure if you will make any difference. Furthermore, the team lacks clarity on their roles and responsibilities, and there are disagreements among members.

To improve productivity and foster a healthy team spirit, what steps can you take to ensure progress towards the project objectives?

See Author's suggestion on page 195–196.

Notes

1 "What is Global Health?" *Duke Global Health Institute*, accessed March 21, 2023, https://globalhealth.duke.edu/what-global-health
2 Gareth Jones and Jennifer George, *Essentials of Contemporary Management*, 6th edn, (New York: McGraw-Hill Education, 2009), 10.
3 Jeffrey Krivis, "Can We Call a Truce? Ten Tips for Negotiating Workplace Conflicts," *Mediate.com* (2017), https://mediate.com/can-we-call-a-truce-ten-tips-for-negotiating-workplace-conflicts/
4 "How to Handle Conflict in the Workplace," last modified January 5, 2018, accessed April 1, 2023, https://blink.ucsd.edu/HR/supervising/conflict/handle.html#8.-Build-on-your-success

References

Duke Global Health Institute. "What is Global Health?" Accessed March 21, 2023. https://globalhealth.duke.edu/what-global-health

Jones, Gareth R. and Jennifer M. George. *Essentials of Contemporary Management*. New York: McGraw-Hill Education. 2009.

Krivis, Jeffrey. "Can We Call a Truce? Ten Tips for Negotiating Workplace Conflicts." *Mediate.com*. https://mediate.com/can-we-call-a-truce-ten-tips-for-negotiating-workplace-conflicts/

University of California San Diego. "How to Handle Conflict in the Workplace." *Blink*. Last modified January 5, 2018. https://blink.ucsd.edu/HR/supervising/conflict/handle.html#8.-Build-on-your-success

3 Developing detailed activity plans

Following approval of the project proposal and signing of the funding agreement with the implementing partner (either the government's MOH or an NGO), a multitude of tasks are initiated simultaneously. The PM is often inundated with various activities including recruitment and deployment of staff, procurement of project items such as computers, vehicles, and building materials, organization of staff training, participation in meetings, conducting site visits, budget development, and many other responsibilities, all at the same time. During such a busy startup phase, the PM may struggle to develop a comprehensive plan outlining the tasks the team members will undertake. In the absence of such a detailed plan however, the project cannot proceed smoothly in an organized manner.

Not having a detailed plan of project activities is not an option. As Sir Winston Churchill once said, *"He who fails to plan is planning to fail."* This statement proves true, especially in project management. The absence of a practical plan of action can lead to a chaotic start of a health project leading to confusion among team members. This can demoralize them, especially if they do not see the logical arrangement of project tasks. In the absence of a detailed and cohesive plan of activities, they may end up carrying out tasks haphazardly. This hinders the progress of the project.

> During my visits to various project locations, I noticed stockout issues with medicines and supplies multiple times during the life of a project. This was mainly due to the lack of a comprehensive detailed plan, particularly in terms of ordering and purchasing the supplies in sufficient quantities and at the appropriate time. However, some of these project teams eventually learned to develop and implement detailed protocols, assigning specific team members to handle the procurement of medical supplies and ensuring the plan was followed. The stockout of supplies was no longer an issue for these projects.

DOI: 10.4324/9781003405245-4

Purpose and documentation of activity plans

Creating a detailed work plan is essential in ensuring project activities are carried out in a logical and sequential order. By developing this plan early on, the PM and their team members can easily visualize the sequence and timeline of activities from the project's inception. Documenting the plan also enables the PM to share it with the team members, organizational senior management, and external stakeholders. This widespread dissemination helps promote transparency and garner support from all those involved in the project's implementation, funding, approval, and evaluation.

There exist various names for this type of work plan, such as a 'detailed implementation plan,' a 'detailed plan of action,' or a 'detailed work plan,' etc. Some organizations prefer the term 'logical framework' or 'logframe,' while others use 'results framework.' 'Bar (or Gantt) chart' is another format. 'Critical Path Analysis' is yet another way of documenting project activity plans. The MOH may have its own standard format for recording its plans for project activities. Despite some variations in format, the one fundamental purpose of these plans is to map out the detailed steps a project will undertake to execute its activities and sub-activities.

Throughout this book we use the term 'Detailed Activity Plan,' or DAP as mentioned in Chapter 1, which can be presented in a simple hand-drawn table or a more sophisticated and comprehensive computer-generated flowchart. Various computer programs can generate visual flowcharts and tables. For simplicity, one can utilize a simple hand-made tabular format using either flip chart papers and marker pens, or a table in a computer spreadsheet. We prefer to keep the DAP simple and present its creation in a tabular format.

Besides being an activity guide, the DAP document acts as a checklist for the health project team to ensure all the activities and sub-activities are implemented as planned. The PM and their team members use the work plan to monitor their project progress for themselves. The DAP often serves as a requirement for the funding agency's decision-making process.[1] By contributing to the creation of a work plan and understanding their respective roles, team members can greatly increase team spirit and ensure the timely completion of the project.

The DAP outlines in detail what activities the project is to do, how to do them, who will be responsible for doing or overseeing each activity, when will each activity start and finish, and a few other related information such as assumptions and risks. The essential elements of a DAP are the *What, How, Who, When, Risks, Assumptions,* and *Notes* relating to project tasks and sub-tasks. The project team can create a DAP using a table with columns and rows and following a six-step guide detailed below.

Steps for developing a DAP

Step 1 Analyzing project interventions and activities

The project proposal, approved by both the funding agency and organizational management, will only provide a general overview of the interventions and major activities involved. Due to page limitations, proposals are not expected to provide extensive details. However, an ideal DAP is a more comprehensive document that concentrates on the project's tasks and sub-tasks.

As a first step, the project team must carefully examine the project proposal and identify all the interventions and activities that will be carried out. A project aimed at improving children's health may contain multiple interventions listed in the proposal. The DAP needs to consider each of these interventions, which could include for example, malaria control for young children, reducing occurrences of diarrheal episodes among children, providing proper treatment for childhood pneumonia, and deworming children, among others. These interventions are intended to improve the health of children in the project communities and are likely already included in the approved proposal.

The project team needs to list in the DAP all the interventions and all the major activities under each intervention. As an illustration, we will focus only on the intervention of malaria control among young children. There are multiple activities that the project team can do to reduce malaria among children. Major ones may already be outlined in the project proposal.

Step 2 Listing all major activities that the project will undertake

In developing the DAP, the team must carefully think through the activities that are appropriate and feasible, and list these in the DAP document. Table 3.1 lists five selected activities under the malaria control intervention.

Table 3.1 Intervention and activities

Intervention	Activity (Task)
Malaria control in children under 5 years of age	1. Distribution of long-lasting insecticide-treated nets (LLINs)
	2. Residual indoor spraying
	3. Removal or destruction of mosquito breeding sites
	4. Supply of malaria rapid diagnostic test kits (RDTs) to village health workers
	5. Supply of anti-malarial drugs to health centers

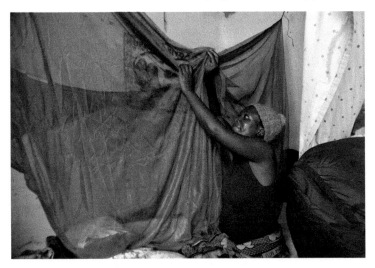

Image 3.1 Setting up malaria bed net at home in Tanzania
Credit: Riccardo Gangale

Let us focus on one important activity related to this intervention for our discussion - the distribution of LLINs to prevent malaria, which is Activity (Task) # 1 in Table 3.1.

Especially in malaria zones the LLINs should be used by everyone, especially young children. Their immune system, not being fully mature yet, is unprepared to fight malaria. Thus, there is a high malaria mortality rate among young children. UNICEF estimates that globally a child dies from malaria every two minutes,[2] and it describes LLINs as the most effective prevention tool against malaria.[3] Image 3.1 shows a mother setting up a mosquito bed net at home to protect her children from malaria.

Step 2 then answers the question "*What* will the project do under the malaria control intervention?"

As we move forward with the development of the DAP, we will expand on this table. For the sake of brevity we will consider those DAP elements that only relate to Activity # 1 in the following discussion.

Step 3 Listing all sub-activities under each activity

In this step the team will proceed with the planning for a number of sub-activities (or sub-tasks) related to each activity (task) outlined in the DAP. Using the example of the distribution of LLINs, which is Activity (Task) # 1 in Table 3.1, the team will need to plan multiple sub-tasks that will lead to Task 1.

Step 3 in the DAP process involves breaking down each task into smaller sub-tasks. This helps to clarify the specific steps that the project team will take to complete each activity outlined in Step 2. Thus, while the activities in the plan show *What* is to be done (Step 2), the sub-activities or sub-tasks (in this Step 3) show *How* the project team will accomplish each of these activities.

To distribute LLINs, several errands must be taken in a specific sequence. First, it may be necessary to hold a meeting with community leaders in the project area to inform them of the distribution and obtain their approval. Education sessions for children's caregivers would likely be organized by the health project to teach them about the benefits of the nets and provide information about the distribution date and location. Procurement staff must also order the LLINs from the vendor or manufacturer with ample lead time before the actual distribution. Other errands may include arranging storage in a warehouse and transporting the nets to the distribution sites, and preparing logbooks to record distribution and collect signatures from recipients. These efforts are all sub-tasks that must be completed to ensure successful distribution, which is the task or the activity under consideration.

In this step we focus on five specific sub-tasks shown in Table 3.2. These five sub-tasks are: meeting with community leaders; organizing health education sessions; ordering and procuring the LLINs; storing and transporting these bednets to the distribution sites, and finally, distributing the nets to the community members.

Table 3.2 Activity and its sub-activities

Activity (Task)	Sub-activity (Sub-task)
1. Distribution of LLINs	1.1. Meet with community leaders
	1.2. Organize education sessions for caregivers on malaria prevention with bed nets
	1.3. Order LLINs from vendor; complete the purchase and receive the nets at project warehouse
	1.4. Store nets in project warehouse; arrange transportation of the bed nets to distribution sites
	1.5. Distribute the LLINs to the caregivers
2. Residual indoor spraying	
3. Removal or destruction of mosquito breeding sites	
4. Supply of malaria rapid diagnostic test kits (RDTs) to village health workers	
5. Supply of anti-malarial drugs to health centers	

In developing the actual DAP a team can further break down each of these sub-tasks into their finer components, and plan for those even more detailed sub-tasks as well. To keep this illustration simple however, we only focus on the first level sub-task.

Step 4: Specifying who will be responsible for each sub-task

This step of DAP development assigns team members the responsibility to complete each task and sub-task. The *job title* of the selected team members is mentioned alongside every sub-task in the DAP document to indicate the designated person for the sub-task. This individual is either the one who completes that sub-task, or functions as a point person (also known as Point of Contact) for that particular sub-task. It is mandatory for every sub-task to have a designated point person. The point person normally does not necessarily execute the sub-task alone, but functions as the 'go to' person that has information about the sub-task. This means, as several individuals carry out a sub task, the point person leads and guides them, gives them information, and receives information from them related to their work. The PM depends on the point persons for information and advice about their respective sub-tasks. A point person may also at times be the one to conduct an entire sub-task alone. Table 3.3 illustrates

Table 3.3 Designated team members for sub-tasks

Activity (Task)	Sub-activity (Sub-task)	Point of contact (point person)
1.1. Distribution of LLINs	1.1. Meet with community leaders	1.1. Assistant project manager
	1.2. Organize education sessions for caregivers on malaria prevention with bed nets	1.2. Community health promoter (usually trains and supervises community health workers)
	1.3. Order LLINs from vendor; complete the purchase and receive the nets at project warehouse	1.3. Procurement officer (in charge of purchasing and securing project items).
	1.4. Store nets in project warehouse; arrange transportation of the bed nets to distribution sites	1.4. Project warehouse manager (supervises store assistant)
	1.5. Distribute the LLINs to the caregivers	1.5. Project officer (supervises community health promoters)

how the DAP document specifies the person responsible for each sub-task. Step 4 then answers the question *"Who* will be the responsible person for specific sub-tasks?"

Appendix B gives an illustrative format of a basic DAP for a child immunization project. You will notice there is no separate column for writing the title of the person responsible for each sub-task or the point person in that format. For saving space in the DAP, this information is sometimes written in the Notes column, where the progress of the project is also noted. The format in Annex B shows this variation.

Step 5: Providing a timeframe for each sub-task.

Each sub-task should have a specific start and end time in the DAP. To achieve this, the team must thoroughly plan out the sequential progression of every sub-task. For instance, the actual distribution of the LLINs should wait until the APM has discussed this with the local community leaders. And the CHPs or CHWs need to educate the mothers and caregivers about the proper use of malaria bed nets before these are distributed to them. Again, the warehousing and transporting of the nets logically must take place after purchasing these from the vendors.

This step shows the project team what sequence they should follow for carrying out each sub-task. Table 3.4 displays the months for each sub-activity on the right-hand column next to the assigned person. For simplicity, this column shows a project timeline starting in January and ending in December. The DAP can also utilize quarters (e.g. Q1, Q2, etc.), with each quarter representing three months of the year.

Thus, Step 5 answers the question, *"When* will the project team conduct each sub-task?"

Sometimes sub-tasks may overlap. For instance, in this illustration, while the process of selecting and buying LLINs (sub-task 1.3) is still ongoing, health education sessions for caregivers (sub-task 1.2) will start. Selecting vendors, purchasing the nets (especially if they are in large volume), and receiving these in the warehouse generally take a considerable amount of time, which is why sub-task 1.3 is planned for six months. However, it is important not to delay the health education sessions. These can start even while the procurement officer is in the final stages of purchasing the LLINs.

The APM has scheduled meetings with community leaders in January and February (note that these months are for illustration only) to inform them of the plan for distributing LLINs. This is sub-task 1.1. It is expected that the leaders will provide their consent. Afterward, vendor selection and net purchase can commence in March and continue

Table 3.4 Timeframe for project sub-activities

Sub-activity (Sub-task)	Point of contact (Point person)	Timeframe											
		J	F	M	A	M	J	J	A	S	O	N	D
1.1. Meet with community leaders	1.1. Assistant project manager	X	X										
1.2. Organize education sessions for caregivers on malaria prevention with bed nets	1.2. Community health promoter (usually trains and supervises community health workers)							X	X	X			
1.3. Order LLINs from vendor; complete the purchase and receive the nets at project warehouse	1.3. Procurement officer (in charge of purchasing and securing project items).			X	X	X	X	X	X				
1.4. Store nets in project warehouse; arrange transportation of the bed nets to distribution sites	1.4. Project warehouse manager (supervises store assistant)								X				
1.5. Distribute the LLINs to the caregivers	1.5. Project officer (supervises community health promoters)									X	X	X	

for six months. Any delay in ordering and purchasing the LLINs will result in a delay in their distribution, potentially causing caregivers to forget what they learn about these bed nets during their health education sessions.

Then there are sub-tasks that must logically take place only after the previous ones are completed. Sub-task 1.4 (storage and transportation of the nets) cannot take place before sub-task 1.3 (ordering nets from vendors) has been completed for obvious reasons.

The above discussion aims to provide a basic illustration. In actuality, the number of activities and sub-activities can be quite large, particularly in complex health projects that encompass a broad range of interventions. However, following a logical, step-by-step approach to DAP development, as outlined above, can help create a practical and efficient plan.

Step 6 Considering assumptions and risks for sub-tasks

The project team relies on certain assumptions regarding project tasks and sub-tasks. For example, the procurement and storage of LLINs is dependent on the availability of a manufacturer or vendor who can supply these in adequate quantities. Therefore, it is necessary to assume that a source for procuring enough LLINs in a timely manner is available.

By listing the project's assumptions in the DAP and sharing the document, one can help both the project team and external stakeholders such as the organization's headquarters, local government officials, and funding bodies to better appreciate the critical dependencies and difficulties of the project's tasks and sub-tasks. The assumptions outline the necessary conditions that need to be in place for the project to successfully complete its planned sub-tasks. For instance, in our example of distributing LLINs, the project's success depends on the manufacturer or vendor's ability to produce and supply the required number of nets on time.

When creating a DAP, it is important to consider and document potential risks that could hinder project activities and sub-activities. For instance, if there is widespread flooding in the project area, it could create a major obstacle to completing project work. This could affect sub-tasks such as organizing health education for caregivers or distributing bed nets. In some cases, entire communities may be submerged under water for days. If this type of flooding happens frequently, such as those that occur in certain regions of the world, it is important for the project team to acknowledge this potential risk in the DAP document.

Thus, it is crucial to include in the DAP a comprehensive list of assumptions and risks that may affect important sub-tasks. These should be presented in a column after the timeframe. However, simply listing them is not enough. It is equally important to identify how these challenges will be addressed and mitigated. For instance, if the manufacturer or vendor is unable to supply the project with the required number of LLINs within the stipulated timeframe, team members should consider alternative options. Would it be wise to seek multiple manufacturers and vendors who can provide the LLINs if one fails? Alternatively, could the team procure the nets from various suppliers, each producing and shipping a small quantity of nets instead of relying solely on one source for a large shipment?

For mitigating the risks that negatively affect project progress, the team would want to plan alternative strategies in advance. For instance, if flooding is a seasonal event during the rainy months, then the project team can plan tasks and sub-tasks (such as the malaria education sessions and actual distribution of the LLINs) for those months when flooding is less likely.

To create a more comprehensive and practical DAP document, alternate or mitigation plans should be documented in a separate column under 'Notes,' alongside the team's considerations of assumptions and risks. This column can also include other important information related to sub-tasks.

It is important to note that assumptions and risks within the control of the project team should not be included in the DAP. For example, stating that staff will receive training for giving the community members effective malaria education sessions is not a valid assumption. It is rather an expectation. Similarly, potential problems that can be avoided or resolved by the project team, such as the inability to secure a storage facility for LLINs, should not be considered a risk factor. Risks and assumptions are *external* factors beyond the control of the project, such as unexpected weather or climate issues, political, or economic changes.

Step 6 answers the question, "What are the assumptions and risks that the health project might encounter? And how will it address these?"

Other DAP elements

In certain DAPs, there is supplementary information included. Within the DAP document, project teams may outline targets, indicators, and means of verification. Although there could be additional elements incorporated into the DAP, we will now turn only to these three.

Targets

In the DAP, each sub-task is assigned a target. The target specifies the amount of work that needs to be completed for a specific sub-task in the project. For example, if the sub-task is to organize health education sessions in the community, the target may be 100 sessions for the entire project duration. This lets the team know that they must conduct 100 health education sessions in the community by the end of the project. Another target could be the distribution of 500 bed nets in the second year of the project. In a DAP document a column to the right of the list of sub-activities may be an appropriate place for including their specific targets.

Indicators

Often DAPs include indicators for sub-activities. One example of an indicator is 'Meeting held with community leaders' for the sub-task of meeting with community leaders. Another example is 'LLINs purchased.' These indicators are very helpful in monitoring and evaluating health projects. The success of the project is measured by the stated indicators, which serve as 'yardsticks.' When monitoring or evaluating a project, it is important to confirm that the tasks and sub-tasks have been completed by utilizing these indicators (yardsticks).

Means of verification

Along with the targets and indicators the 'means of verification' is also quite useful to plan for and include in the DAP document. This helps the project team decide on the sources of information they will use to track progress for each sub-task and its indicator. For instance, to monitor and evaluate the meetings with community leaders, a community leaders meeting logbook can be used. This logbook records important details such as the dates and locations of the meetings, names of attendees, meeting minutes, key decisions, and other relevant information. Such a logbook becomes the source or *means of verification* for that particular sub-task, and some DAP documents have a column specifically for listing these means of verification alongside the indicator column.

Participatory process for developing a DAP

The DAP, as its name suggests, is a highly detailed plan that can be complex, particularly for larger projects with multiple objectives and interventions. Engaging the health project team in the development of the DAP is strongly recommended as it is the most efficient approach to creating such a comprehensive plan utilizing a participatory process.

When team members contribute to crafting the DAP, they become committed to following it. Participation of all the team members helps the PM gain a wider perspective on the DAP. Grappling with challenges and finding the best course of action should not be a burden for the PM alone. This becomes a shared responsibility for the team if they participate in the DAP planning process.

When it comes to contributing to the DAP process, those who are directly involved in the project tasks and sub-tasks should have the most input. However, even those who indirectly support the project, for example, a logistics officer who ensures staff members have transportation to carry out their duties, can also offer valuable insights. People outside of the health project team, such as the MEAL staff, finance officers or the HR manager, may not be directly involved in the health project's day-to-day operations, but it is important to invite them to participate so they appreciate its strategies and contribute to its success. By ensuring that all participants have a clear understanding of the project goals and activities, the PM can gain their support and increase the likelihood of success.

Workshop format

Engaging individuals in the DAP planning process is best achieved through the dynamic format of a workshop. Through small group discussions, large group presentations, and output generation, participants actively contribute to a plan that everyone agrees upon.

During the workshop, individuals use sticky note pads to jot down ideas, create tables and diagrams on flip charts, and present their small group outputs to the larger group using slides or posters. See Images 3.2 and 3.3.

A DAP workshop is usually led by an experienced facilitator, who can be an advisor or a consultant either from within or outside the implementing agency. Alternatively, an experienced PM can also perform the role of a facilitator. The workshop facilitator systematically guides the team through the steps outlined in the sub-section above, 'Steps for Developing a DAP.'

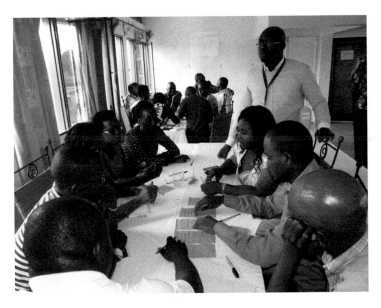

Image 3.2 Small group work at a DAP workshop in Burundi

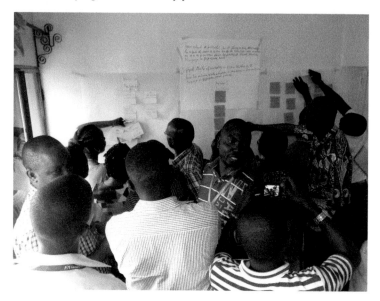

Image 3.3 Workshop participants using flip chart papers and sticky notes to
develop a DAP in Burundi

The experienced facilitator uses different participatory methodologies to conduct the workshop.

Using the DAP developing steps in a workshop.

First, the participants need to get a thorough understanding of what the health project is supposed to do and achieve. They may study materials prepared for this purpose and learn more about their project activities from large group presentations. This is Step 1 above.

The subsequent steps in a DAP workshop involve brainstorming in small groups to choose activities and sub-activities, as discussed above. The ideas from the small groups are then presented to the large group, where everyone gets an opportunity to compare, modify, and accept them. The participants then determine the point of contact for each sub-activity and agree on the timeframe for each one. They also discuss assumptions and risk factors and choose strategies to address them.

Once all the components of the DAP are assembled by the participants in small and large group processes, the draft DAP document is presented for assessment by the PM and other relevant parties.

Necessary adjustments may be made during this phase, after which the DAP is finalized as the project team's work plan.

Involving external stakeholders

To ensure the success of the health project, it is important to consider the impact of external stakeholders beyond the health project team and the implementing organization. Inviting community leaders, MOH representatives, project partner organizations, and funding agencies to participate in the DAP workshop can be highly beneficial. Community leaders are key influencers in the locality where the health project operates, and their understanding and approval are essential for carrying out tasks and sub-tasks. MOH representatives can provide valuable input in selecting project sub-tasks and timeframes, as well as sharing government perspectives and priorities. Partnering agencies and funding organizations may also have valuable insights to share.

The PM should give these external participants appropriate roles in the workshop process. Even if they can only attend an opening session, their presence is important and adds validity to the DAP. For example, an MOH official may simply give an opening remark or share health priorities for the government, while a funding organization's representative may share rules and regulations on financial matters. The PM must not hesitate to invite specialists and advisors from their own or partner organizations as they may have valuable ideas to contribute.

Key takeaways

- Developing a DAP is essential in the very early stages of project implementation.
- A project DAP is useful in many ways:
  - It guides team members to conduct project tasks and sub-tasks.
  - Funding agencies often make decisions based on the DAP.
  - It functions as a checklist for the project team to monitor progress and to evaluate the project.
  - The participatory process for developing DAP fosters team spirit.
- A project team can utilize six basic steps to develop a DAP. These steps help to document the DAP plan to show the *What, How, Who, When, Risks, Assumptions* and Notes that relate to the project tasks and sub-tasks. The DAP document may contain additional features such as targets, indicators, and means of verification.
- A participatory workshop format for developing the DAP is ideal.
- External stakeholders can make significant contributions to the DAP planning process and the project team should include them in a DAP workshop.

Discussion questions

1. What are the potential problems of not developing a DAP early in the project cycle?
2. What are the six basic steps for developing a DAP? Briefly describe each step.
3. What is the advantage of inviting external stakeholders to a DAP workshop?
4. Discuss the importance of including in the DAP document a set of assumptions and risks for each sub-task.
5. Multiple choice questions. Circle the number of the correct answer.

   5.1. The purpose of developing a DAP is to:

      5.1.1. Report the financial status of the project to the donors.
      5.1.2. Let the organizational management know of project problems.
      5.1.3. Articulate what activities the project will undertake and how it will do them.
      5.1.4. Replace the project proposal with an alternative implementation plan.

   5.2 As a first step for developing a DAP one should:

      5.2.1. Review project budget to see the total amount of funding available.
      5.2.2. Create small and large groups to participate in the DAP workshop.
      5.2.3. Create a list of team members who will serve as point persons for project activities.
      5.2.4. Carefully review the project proposal to see what interventions have been planned.

   5.3. A DAP workshop is useful:

      5.3.1. When only the PM facilitates the workshop.
      5.3.2. If participants share their views in small and large groups.
      5.3.3. When participants do not waste time studying first the project interventions.
      5.3.4. If there is no assumption made relating to the sub-tasks.

   5.4. An acceptable assumption statement in a DAP document would be:

      5.4.1. The project will teach community members how to prevent the spread of COVID-19 when they visit health centers for receiving services.

5.4.2. The project's health promoter will train community health workers on how to give nutrition education to caregivers of children.

5.4.3. The MOH will supply an adequate number of vaccine doses to the health centers that the project supports.

5.4.4. The project's site supervisor will make regular site visits to monitor health center construction.

See correct answers on page 194.

Case study exercise

After completing your university education, imagine you have accepted a PM position in an LMIC where resources are limited. Your project is in its initial stages and there are numerous start-up activities that require your attention. You have realized that organizing a planning workshop and the DAP document creation is essential and must be done quickly, but you have limited time to focus on it. What steps can you take to ensure that the DAP is developed while you attend to other important project matters?

See Author's suggestion on page 196.

Notes

1 Andrew Green, *An Introduction to Health Planning for Developing Health Systems* (Oxford: Oxford University Press, 2007).
2 "Ten facts about mosquito nets you didn't know," UNICEF South Sudan, last modified November 5, 2020, accessed April 8, 2023, www.unicef.org/southsudan/stories/ten-facts-about-mosquito-nets-you-didnt-know
3 "Fighting malaria with long-lasting insecticidal nets (LLINs)," UNICEF Supply Division, last modified February 5, 2022, accessed April 8, 2023, www.unicef.org/supply/stories/fighting-malaria-long-lasting-insecticidal-nets-llins

References

Green, A. (2007). *An Introduction to Health Planning for Developing Health Systems*. Oxford University Press.
UNICEF South Sudan. 2020. "Ten facts about mosquito nets you didn't know." Last modified November 5. www.unicef.org/southsudan/stories/ten-facts-about-mosquito-nets-you-didnt-know
UNICEF Supply Division. 2022. "Fighting malaria with long-lasting insecticidal nets (LLINs)." Last modified February 5. www.unicef.org/supply/stories/fighting-malaria-long-lasting-insecticidal-nets-llins

4 Improving project team performance

In the last two chapters, we explored the process of building a global health project team and developing a detailed plan of activities for the team members. As the team starts to operate the project according to the DAP, the PM may notice that not all the project team members possess the same level of expertise. Some individuals may have experience from previous work, while others may find the project activities unfamiliar and challenging, particularly if they lack professional training.

> As a global health professional, I started my career in a rural area of Bangladesh right after completing my university course in the USA. I was responsible for managing a health project that aimed to improve the health of young children in a resource-constrained area of the country.
>
> This was a new project, and as a new PM, I was struggling to decide which activity the team should start with. Fortunately, I had a senior staff member on my team who had experience as a trainer. He had already prepared a training plan for the project staff just before I joined as the PM. I had him start training the junior staff, and soon, all project staff completed their orientation and training.
>
> Through this experience, I learned that orienting and training project staff is one of the first steps project leadership should undertake. The project has officially started; the clock is ticking, and there is little time to waste! Your implementing organization is depending on project success; the local government health officials are keen to see the project supporting them; and the donor organization would soon expect results from their investment in the project.

Once the project begins, it is necessary to orient the team members to the project activities immediately and continue improving their capacity with periodic training, coaching, mentoring, and incentivizing.

DOI: 10.4324/9781003405245-5

Orientation of project staff

The PM must ensure that all team members have a shared understanding of project goals, objectives, and activities, regardless of their current skill level. Furthermore, the PM has specific expectations of the team's approach to project activities, which the team should become aware of. Any uneven levels of understanding among team members about the project can impede team collaboration and productivity. Therefore, it is imperative that the team receives a consistent orientation.

The PM or an experienced facilitator (e.g., consultants or senior staff from the country, regional, or international headquarters) should lead the orientation sessions to ensure success for the project team. It is crucial that the PM or the facilitator first reviews important project documents, such as the project proposal, DAP, baseline survey report, and relevant government policies and agreements to become familiar with the project's key objectives.

The orientation should be conducted systematically so that the project team gains a comprehensive understanding of the project's goal, objectives, outcomes, outputs, activities, and sub-activities. To illustrate the interrelation of project goals, objectives, and outcomes during the staff orientation session, a diagram similar to the illustrative one in Figure 4.1 can be shared with the team in a PowerPoint slide.

Besides project goal, objectives, and outcomes the orientation session should cover project outputs, activities, and sub-activities as well, which do not appear in this figure.

There are specific activities that the team members will undertake to operate a health project. For instance, some team members may be

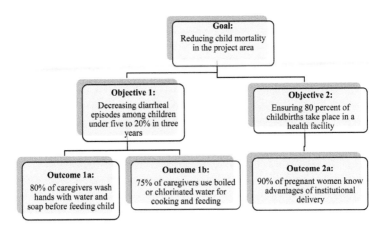

Figure 4.1 Illustrative summary of the project goal, objectives, and outcomes

responsible for educating community mothers and caregivers about the importance of handwashing with soap. The educating of mothers and caregivers is an activity (task). This task may involve using visuals, such as printed flip books or demonstrating the actual handwashing using water and soap. Using the flip book and giving the handwashing demo are considered sub-activities (sub-tasks) that should be carried out at the appropriate time during the education session.

To ensure consistency across all project sites, the handwashing education session should be conducted in a uniform manner. This could involve weekly gatherings of the caregivers of children for health education sessions. Additionally, there may be weekly radio or TV broadcasts of health messages that community members can tune into. Staff members responsible for organizing these tasks and sub-tasks should have a clear understanding of the contents, place, frequency, and other pertinent information. The staff orientation sessions cover each task and sub-task of the project.

During the outbreak of the ebola virus disease (EVD) in a neighboring country in 2018, a health project in South Sudan began an interactive radio broadcast program discussing EVD prevention. Community members received prevention messages through these radio sessions, and they called in to ask questions and requested clarifications. Trained project staff made these radio broadcasts and answered questions.

The same project also organized 'street theaters' at project sites to improve EVD prevention knowledge and practice in the communities. A local drama troupe performed skits in open air streetside 'theaters' to demonstrate the transmission and prevention of EVD in the communities. A similar street performance is depicted in Image 4.1.

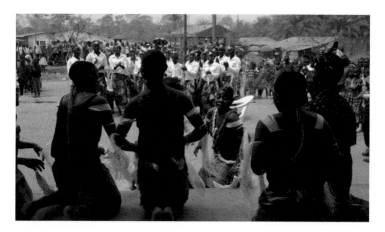

Image 4.1 Street drama in Cameroon
Credit: Garviston

These kinds of tasks are quite complicated, which the team meticulously prepares for, and undertakes. How these tasks and sub-tasks will be carried out, who will be responsible for which tasks, what are the problems that should be anticipated and how these problems would be addressed, are all critical areas that the project team needs to understand during the orientation sessions.

Additionally, the PM should use this orientation time to define their expectations regarding team productivity and standards. For example, the PM may want to have a written report by certain deadline on key activities that the team performs. Deadlines allow the PM to monitor project progress in a timely manner and write their own routine reports. Or they might set a rule that site activities ought to be completed at a specific time of day, with the teams returning to the project office by a certain hour each evening. This type of time setting is especially important in dangerous locations where there is conflict or violence between groups of people. The orientation sessions give the PM the opportunity to set these expectations and rules for the team.

Depending on the volume of activities and complexity of the project, several well-planned orientation sessions may be necessary to prepare the team adequately for the project tasks.

Periodic training of team members

Some PMs may have the mindset that team members come with adequate training and knowledge, and they do not need additional training. But experience shows team members need periodic training to keep their skills sharp. The PM must ensure all team members have adequate training on the tasks and sub-tasks they are supposed to perform.

While orientation sessions instruct project staff about what to do, who should do which part, when they should do these tasks and so forth, the *training* of project staff helps them to learn *how* to do these tasks.

Training can cover several areas, but two important types of tasks that staff should be trained in are broadly, *administrative* and *technical* in nature.

Administrative

There are a number of administrative tasks that project staff need to do. Filling out forms, checking inventory, selecting vendors and contractors, and clocking time, are only a few examples of administrative tasks.

During administrative training specific forms or papers should be introduced and instructions given as to how team members will use these for documenting information. Staff should receive training on protocols that they need to maintain (e.g., per diem that staff members receive before a site visit should not exceed a certain amount, and they must draw the funds a specific number of days before their trip).

Moreover, the project staff must comply with the rules and regulations set by the government and donor organizations. These guidelines may involve avoiding specific geographical locations due to political or security reasons and implementing a transparent bidding process when awarding contracts to vendors and suppliers. Thus, it is the responsibility of the PM to ensure that team members receive detailed training on these administrative procedures and practices at the beginning of the project cycle.

Technical

When you assume the role of the PM, you are ultimately responsible for ensuring that your project staff receives the necessary technical training. However, it is not required that you personally provide this training. Your organization's headquarters, regional or country offices may have qualified trainers or advisors available to train your team members in specific technical areas. Project partner organizations may also have trainers that they can offer for training the team. If you possess the technical knowledge and experience to train your staff or data collectors to conduct evaluations for instance, then you should do so. However, it is important to carefully consider your training responsibilities and ensure that you have enough time to fulfill your daily PM duties.

In the field of global health, there are established technical strategies and standards that are commonly followed for various activities. Each country's MOH has specific protocols for health care services such as administering childhood vaccines and deworming medications. The preparation of ORS solution follows a specific method. For pregnant women, there are a specific number of required ANC visits at a health center for them to receive necessary pregnancy-related services. The project team needs to know these norms. Technical training is crucial in equipping project staff with the knowledge and skills to perform their tasks in accordance with accepted standards.

Even project staff that received training in a previous work setting may find that some of their skills have become rusty over time, or that they need to upgrade their skills as new innovative approaches in global health programming are adopted. For instance, paper-based questionnaires were commonly used in project surveys in the past, but nowadays, hand-held devices like smartphones or tablets are increasingly replacing them. Therefore, staff responsible for data collection in surveys will need to learn how to use these relatively advanced tools and strategies.

Furthermore, the PM can expect staff turnover as team members leave, and new individuals join the team as the project progresses. Therefore, it is essential for the PM to ensure that all team members receive sufficient training to carry out their project activities using the best practices in global health. The following are key steps one should follow to ensure effective team training.

Training needs assessment

Before commencing any training, it is important to conduct a thorough training needs assessment. This helps identify and document any gaps in staff performance, providing the PM with valuable insights into the areas that require training. The training can then be tailored to address these gaps, ensuring that it is relevant and beneficial in enhancing staff output where there is a deficiency.

Conducting a training needs assessment can be as simple as observing team members' performance, administering a written skills test, or evaluating their practical demonstration of a task. These methods can effectively identify the areas where team members require further training. It is advisable to keep a written record of the results of the needs assessment, which can be used to compare and analyze the improvements made in team capacity over time.

To give an example, when it comes to providing health education to mothers of young children on proper nutrition, it is quite important for staff to incorporate more interactive elements into their sessions. This could include allowing attendees to ask questions, share their own experiences, and engage in other participatory activities. By conducting a thorough training needs assessment, any gaps in knowledge or skills can be identified and targeted training can be provided. In this case of health education sessions, for instance, staff members responsible for organizing them should receive training on participatory adult learning processes.

Selecting training topics based on the needs assessment makes the trainees more likely to stay engaged and energized during their training. Other examples of skills that staff may need to learn or reinforce through training, and which the needs assessment can identify include using audio-visuals correctly during health education sessions, teaching midwives how to use the partograph during childbirth, and showing pharmacy staff how to properly store medicines and supplies in the health center dispensary.

Setting training goals and objectives

To ensure training is productive, both the PM and trainers should set clear goals and objectives for the training based on the results of the

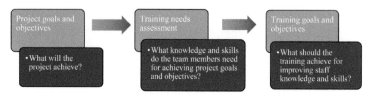

Figure 4.2 Sequential steps from project goals to training needs assessment to training goals

needs assessment. Each training type and session should have specific goals and objectives. A goal for a technical training session for an MNCH project team may be articulated as, "Following the training, the participants will learn to teach midwives at health centers how to implement skin-to-skin contact between the mother and her newborn baby." Another example of a training session goal for team members that improve the health of women in the communities could be, "After completing the training the participants will acquire the knowledge and skills to organize participatory health education sessions for village women."

The goals for training team members should align with the *project's* goals and objectives. As shown in Figure 4.2, project goals and objectives guide the assessment of staff performance, which in turn determines the *training* goals and objectives based on gaps identified in the assessment. The PM must help teammates bridge these gaps through appropriate training to ensure a successful project outcome.

Trainer selection

The PM or senior staff from the headquarters or regional office can serve as the trainer for a particular training. There may be a training officer or advisor within the project team, whose role is to train the team members on technical matters. Sometimes projects run by NGOs contract trained MOH staff to provide such technical training. Many of these government trainers will have received training from the WHO, UNICEF, or other recognized global health organizations. These higher-level trainers are often called 'Master Trainers.' The Master Trainers train junior trainers in the MOH system, who in turn train government staff that work in health facilities and communities. In many LMICs Master Trainers from the MOH are often available to help train NGO staff on technical areas.

A good trainer remains current on the most recent updates related to technical topics. The PM will want to ensure the individual has adequate experience in the adult learning process in addition to having training experience on technical topics. This key requirement equally applies to the implementing organization's in-house trainers just as well as the Master Trainers from the MOH or external training consultants that the project or the implementing organization may recruit.

An effective trainer engages the trainees in a *participatory* process, encouraging everyone to openly share their views, questions, and comments. In selecting the trainer, the PM must find the best individual who not only has the right credentials but also possesses deep experience in training.

In many places trainers rely too heavily on PowerPoint slides during training sessions. Many of them merely read aloud the contents of innumerable slides, making the training session dry and dull for participants. Adult learners require a different approach than the children in a classroom setting. In adult training small group discussions, relevant activities, and engaging simulations are necessary for participant engagement and retention of knowledge.

> In some cases, trainers may use language that is unfamiliar to their trainees. For example, during a visit to a rural health project in a francophone country, I heard about a trainer who used polished French in the PowerPoint slides and lectures during training sessions. However, the trainees were all from village health centers and only spoke their own local dialect, so they could not understand anything being presented. This was a waste of time and project funds, as the training did not benefit anyone. The PM will want to ensure that language barriers are addressed, and appropriate translations are provided to make sure everyone can benefit from the training.

Training preparations

Effective training requires detailed preparations. Working closely with the trainer the PM ensures all necessary training items, including logistics, and per diem for the trainers and participants are in place. For training that is quite involved, one ought to prepare a detailed checklist. The PM may give responsibilities to several of the project team members to go through the checklist and secure all necessary items well in advance of the training.

> As a trainer on a global health project, I have had the opportunity to work with detailed checklists that cover every aspect of the training process. These checklists were divided up among support team members, who meticulously gathered all the necessary items in the checklist to ensure that the training sessions ran smoothly.

One interesting item on the checklist was duct tape. This was used to secure and cover the projector's power cord on the floor to prevent tripping during the training session! The checklist also included whiteboard markers of specific colors, name tags for participants, and even extra projector bulbs in case one burned out during a session!

The level of detail that went into crafting these checklists and organizing the items was impressive. By having everything prepared beforehand, the training sessions became easy to conduct. Working with such well coordinated teammates helped me gain a deeper appreciation for thorough preparations in advance of the actual training.

Announcements about the training and invitations to the training participants must go out sufficiently ahead of time for them to make preparations. Some training might require team members to read certain materials before beginning the actual training. They need to get these materials ahead of the training sessions.

Even in the case of remote or distance learning with online presentations, preparations are necessary. The participants must receive login instructions ahead of time so they can start the online session in a timely manner if it is live training. They may need materials to review and prepare ahead of time. It is useful for someone to connect online with the trainees prior to the actual training session so audio-visual connections can be tested, and problems fixed. This simple step can prevent technical glitches and time wasting during the actual training session.

There are other things to organize before training begins. A training agenda with important information about the sessions, training objectives, room numbers, etc., is useful to share in advance with the trainees. Training venue and logistics including seating arrangements, accommodation and transportation of the participants, snacks and meal arrangements must all be in place before the training starts. Audio-visual equipment, electric fans or air-conditioners, and other such items should be tested prior to the training to ensure they are in working order.

Unfortunately, there have been numerous incidents where training sessions have not gone as planned due to the oversight of minor details by the PM or a delegated staff. For example: seating arrangements have not been suitable, causing the chairs and tables to be rearranged at the start of a session taking up valuable training time; rooms lacked proper lighting or windows; air-conditioning malfunctioned; or microphones failed. To prevent these issues, it is highly recommended for the PM or a team member to personally ensure that all necessary preparations have been made prior to the commencement of training. By using a checklist, surprises and mishaps can be avoided.

Ensuring every detail is taken care of is crucial for successful staff training. During my travels to multiple countries to conduct training for local staff, on many occasions just as I was about to write some-thing during a presentation I discovered the markers I needed for writing on flip charts were all dry! It was disappointing to realize that those responsible for organizing the training had failed to check beforehand on a simple item as the markers. To avoid such mishaps, the PM should ensure that all aspects of the training have been thor-oughly checked.

Refresher training

It is common for team members who received training at the beginning of a project to go through a refresher after a while. With the passage of time knowledge and skills need upgrading.

The refresher training does not have to cover everything in the origi-nal training. Instead, it can focus on the most significant aspects of pro-ject operations. However, new team members should receive the original training and project orientation that the others received at the start of the project.

Due to funding and time constraints, refresher training cannot hap-pen frequently. It is helpful to schedule one at the midpoint of a multi-year project (e.g., around 2.5 years for a five-year project).

All the areas covered above in relation to organizing the initial training, such as types of training, training needs assessment, selection of trainers, training preparations, setting training objectives, and securing training venue and logistics, also apply to refresher training. The PM ought to treat refresher training with the same importance as the initial training.

Training evaluation

When undertaking a major training initiative, whether it is the initial train-ing or a refresher training, it is useful to conduct an evaluation at the end of the training. Reviewing the training activities can assist in improving future training that the project may undertake. It can also aid the imple-menting organization to enrich its training in other projects and locations. The evaluation process contributes to organizational and team learning.

The ideal source for valuable feedback on the training are the partici-pants themselves. A written questionnaire that covers the critical aspects of training, such as training contents, trainer(s) performance, training venue and logistics, can be quite useful for assessing what went well and areas that required improvement.

Also, assessing the knowledge and skill level of the trainees following their training is crucial in gauging the improvements they have made. Some trainers use pre- and post-tests to compare the knowledge and skills of staff before and after the training.

In-service hands-on (practical) training

Training does not always take place in a classroom setting. On-the-job training (OJT) is also beneficial for team members.

Once the PM has trained the project team, assigning them to project sites is the next step. OJT takes place at these project sites where the team members have been placed. Either the PM, or a team member that the PM delegates (ideally those with supervisory roles in the team) should visit the project sites regularly to demonstrate to the staff in a *practical* manner the specific tasks they are to execute.

While performing their job, staff can learn a variety of essential skills as seen in Image 4.2. Examples of such skills may include

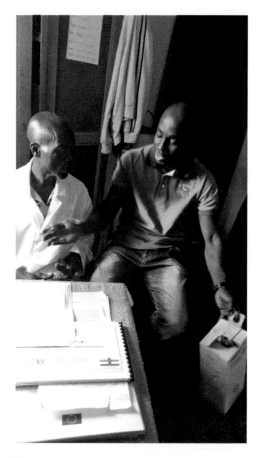

Image 4.2 OJT for nurse at a rural health center on the use of sharps container in Central African Republic

accurately completing registers and logbooks, appropriately storing medicines and supplies in a health center pharmacy, delivering a new-born baby in a health facility, and organizing interactive health education sessions for community members. Note that the OJT is not a substitute for formal classroom instruction, but rather a complementary reinforcement.

Coaching and mentoring of individual team members

In addition to orientation and training the PM may want to arrange coaching and mentoring for certain members of the project team. There may be a few trained staff that need this additional support to perform at an optimal level. Also, the PM may sense the potential among some team members that are ready to assume added responsibilities and may like to promote them to a higher position within the project team. These team members benefit from coaching and mentoring.

Coaching is interacting with team members in a creative process that inspires them to maximize their personal and professional potential.[1] In contrast, mentoring is an arrangement in which a senior or more experienced individual (the mentor) advises, counsels, or guides a junior staff or trainee (i.e., the mentee). The mentor is responsible for providing support to, and constructive feedback on the performance of the mentee placed under their charge. To mentor is to build up the professional capacity of the mentee over a period of time. The mentor takes care not to build up the mentee in his or her own mold, but to allow the mentee to emerge in their own form, only stronger and more competent. The well-known American film director, Steven Spielberg believes, *"The delicate balance of mentoring someone is not creating them in your own image but giving them the opportunity to create themselves."*

There are differences between coaching and mentoring. The Center for Corporate and Professional Development at the Kent State University in Ohio, USA has a valuable set of insights on coaching and mentoring, including a detailed comparison between these two processes. Coaching focuses on specific goals and takes place over a short term (six months to a year). On the other hand, mentoring is a longer-term engagement lasting for a year or more. Coaching improves work output, while mentoring takes a more comprehensive approach focusing on holistic *career development*. Coaching is more structured with scheduled meetings on a weekly, bi-weekly, or monthly basis, while mentoring is more informal, with meetings held as required. Coaching produces *specific and measurable* outcomes, showing improvement in the desired performance areas. Outcomes from a mentoring relationship focuses more on the overall professional growth and development of the mentee without emphasizing specific, measurable results.[2]

The PM can directly function as a coach or a mentor. Alternatively, someone appropriate either inside or outside the organization can serve in that role to support a team member or a group of team members.

Keeping track of all performance improvement activities is important. By diligently documenting the needs, goals, methodology, and outcomes from all types of team capacity improvement efforts, including coaching and mentoring, the PM can monitor the progress made in the team's work outcomes. Documentation is also useful for conducting staff performance appraisals, as well as analyzing and sharing with internal and external audience the data on team capacity improvements.

Incentives and inspiration

Successful PMs often incentivize their team members to increase staff engagement and productivity. Researchists from Harvard University has shown that team members feel most engaged when their PMs show genuine interest in their wellbeing[3] by offering incentives.

Marissa Levin, Founder and CEO of Successful Culture defines an incentive as anything that motivates or encourages individuals to repeat positive behaviors. She maintains, appreciation and positive recognition are the most powerful and sustainable incentives.[4] Incentivizing team members publicly can foster a sense of pride and healthy competition within the team.

The PM can give incentives through various means. Acknowledging outstanding performance of team members with titles such as 'Employee of the Month'; providing them with a complimentary lunch for exceptional work; publicly commending those who have excelled in their tasks; offering attractive perks such as a paid day off; offering opportunities for career advancement within the project team and the organization; and rewarding high-performing team members with bonuses, are all effective incentives and powerful motivators.

To inspire the team so they excel in their project work, the PM should consider implementing the following strategies.[5]

Setting clear goals for the team

Establishing precise and measurable objectives with a defined timeline eliminates any confusion among team members and results in superior work outcomes.

Sharing project vision with the team

To ensure success of the project, the PM needs to communicate their vision clearly and simply to the team. Strong leaders make this a shared vision by demonstrating how every member can contribute to achieving it. When the team buys into the vision, they become more inspired and committed. Equipping and aligning the team with the PM's vision creates a sense of belonging and inspiration to perform at their best.

Empowering and supporting team members

Effective PMs encourage their project team to participate in decision-making. They guide the teammates through discussions to help identify and solve problems. As the project team becomes more competent and confident, the team leader encourages them to independently make decisions and find their own solutions to problems, instead of always relying on the PM to solve them. The team leader must provide their team with the opportunity to innovate and try out new strategies. The team members will appreciate the PM's support as they empower them to do so.

Providing professional growth and development

Fostering the professional growth and development of their team members by seeking out new opportunities for them is an extraordinary talent of the PM. Arranging special courses or training sessions can help develop team members' skills and inspire them to perform better. Sending selected staff to training workshops locally, and in other cities or countries can also foster engagement and loyalty to the project. An exceptional PM takes the time to mentor or coach their team members when necessary to help them grow and advance in their career.

Knowing team members well

Successful leaders take sufficient time to get to know their team members. By attentively listening and learning about each individual in the project team, the PMs stimulate and motivate them. The teammates would want to know that their PM understands their personal traits, knowledge, behaviors, as well as their struggles. This instills confidence in the PM's leadership and inspires the team.

Key takeaways

- The PM is responsible for improving the work output of the project team. They would want to build their team capacity from the earliest stage of project implementation.
- Orientation to the project ensures team members have a good understanding of the project goals, objectives, outcomes, outputs, and activities. It also helps them to learn about the PM's expectations.
- The orientation sessions cover *what* the project staff should do, while the training helps them to learn *how* to do these tasks.
- Training should cover both the administrative and the technical tasks that staff will perform.
- Needs assessments inform the PM about gaps that require specific staff training.
- Training team members can bridge these gaps and improve team accomplishments.
- The trainer must be experienced in adult learning processes besides having adequate *technical* expertise. The PM can serve as a trainer, although usually a training specialist or consultant is hired to train project staff.
- Besides pre-service training the in-service OJT is also beneficial for team members.
- Sometimes the PM detects the need for coaching and mentoring and organizes this additional support for selected members of the project team. There are differences between coaching and mentoring.
- Keeping track of all training activities helps the PM to conduct staff performance appraisals, analyze and report on team capacity improvements, and demonstrate project progress to internal and external audiences.

Discussion questions

1. Why is refresher training important for project team members?
2. Why is it important to link the project goals and objectives with the training goals and objectives?
3. What are the key differences between coaching and mentoring?
4. Table 4.1 contains seven numbered items covered in this chapter, with short descriptions in the right column. However, these descriptions are not arranged in the correct order and do not match the items on the left. Match each numbered item to its description on the right and correctly write the corresponding letter of the description in the middle column.

Table 4.1 Multiple choice questions

Match the following with the answers in the last column	Insert letter of the correct answer	Answer
1. On-the-Job Training		A. Can be achieved through professional growth and development of team members.
2. Mentoring		B. Short term support with specific, measurable outcomes
3. Orientation		C. Necessary for staff to learn the details of how project activities should be done
4. Motivation		D. Can support team members for their career development
5. Coaching		E. Covers basic features of a project, but does not teach how to do specific activities
6. Training		F. Takes place to demonstrate to team members how they should perform specific tasks at their place of work
7. Incentive		G. Can improve staff engagement and productivity

See correct answers on page 194.

Case study exercise

Meet Girma, a valuable member of your health project team in Ethiopia who takes his responsibilities seriously and tries to accomplish his tasks well. However, Girma struggles with meeting deadlines, which affects the project's timely delivery of outputs. Most often he is late turning in reports, making important phone calls, and submitting requests for pharmaceutical supplies needed for the health centers.

He complains he has too many things to do, which prevents him from finishing his tasks on time. As the PM you have observed, Girma is sincere in his efforts but lacks the organizational skills needed to plan and execute tasks efficiently. He doesn't maintain a calendar or prioritize tasks, leading him to be reactive rather than proactive.

How can you help Girma improve his performance? What do you think he needs for improving his organizational skills? How will you arrange this?

See Author's suggestion on page 196–197.

Notes

1 Drawn from the definition of coaching used by the International Coaching Federation.
"What is Coaching," *International Coaching Federation,* accessed October 18, 2022, https://coachingfederation.org/about#:~:text=What%20 is%20Coaching%3F

2 The discussion on the differences between coaching and mentoring is adapted from the Kent State University webpage: Zust, C. (2017, July 5). *Know the difference between Coaching and Mentoring.* Kent State University: The Center for Corporate and Professional Development. www.kent.edu/ yourtrainingpartner/know-difference-between-coaching-and-mentoring

3 Schwartz, T. (2012, January 23). "Why Appreciation Matters So Much." *Harvard Business Review.* https://hbr.org/2012/01/why-appreciation-matters-so-mu.html

4 Levin, M. (2018, September 7). *How to Set up Incentives to Motivate and Bring Out the Best in Your People.* Inc. www.inc.com/marissa-levin/6-strategies-for-implementing-successful-incentives-to-engage-motivate-your-people. html

5 The discussion on strategies for inspiring project teams is drawn from a blog written by Ankit Raiyani. Raiyani, A. (2021, February 17). *7 Key-Steps to Motivate and Inspire Your Team.* LinkedIn. https://www.linkedin.com/ pulse/7-key-steps-motivate-inspire-your-team-ankit-raiyani/

References

Levin, M. 2018. "How to Set up Incentives to Motivate and Bring Out the Best in Your People." *Inc.* Last modified September 7. www.inc.com/marissa-levin/ 6-strategies-for-implementing-successful-incentives-to-engage-motivate-your-people.html

Raiyani, A. 2021. "7 Key-Steps to Motivate and Inspire Your Team." LinkedIn. Last modified February 17. https://www.linkedin.com/pulse/7-key-steps-motivate-inspire-your-team-ankit-raiyani/

Schwartz, T. 2012. "Why Appreciation Matters So Much." *Harvard Business Review.* Last modified January 23. https://hbr.org/2012/01/why-appreciation-matters-so-mu.html

"What is Coaching," *International Coaching Federation,* accessed Oct. 18, 2022, https://coachingfederation.org/about#:~:text=What%20is%20Coaching%3F

Zust, C. 2017. "Know the difference between Coaching and Mentoring." *Kent State University: The Center for Corporate and Professional Development.* Last modified July 5. www.kent.edu/yourtrainingpartner/know-difference-between-coaching-and-mentoring

5 Supervising project team members

In Chapter 2 you have seen that staff supervision is an important component of team building. It is also one of the leadership functions that the PM exercises. Here we discuss the details of this important function of a PM.

Supportive supervision

Management literature provides various descriptions for staff supervision. However, for effectively managing a global health team, the definition given by the Scottish Social Services Council seems to be most appropriate. It states, "*Supervision is a process that involves a manager meeting regularly and interacting with workers(s) to review their work.*"[1]

This definition indicates that the PM must meet with their teammates regularly to interact with them and review their performance. During these meetings, the PM can observe and discuss how their teammates perform their tasks and provide feedback related to their work. It is critical however, that the team members are able to act on the feedback they receive from their PM.

During these interactions the team members should get opportunities to share their perspectives on the project tasks. Listening to their difficulties, ideas, suggestions, and perceptions of their own performance is important for successful supervision. It is a two-way interaction that requires the PM to utilize effective communication skills, both verbal and non-verbal, especially in multicultural settings. When the PM gives feedback that is respectful and understandable, team members are readily motivated to accept it and act on it.

When the feedback is meant to support the team to excel in their work and attain their goals and targets the PM practices *supportive supervision*, which involves working collaboratively with the team to improve their performance and solve any issues that may arise. Instead of 'policing'

DOI: 10.4324/9781003405245-6

them and looking for faults in an authoritarian approach to supervision, the PM acts as a teacher, coach, or mentor, building strong relationships while focusing on performance improvement. By practicing supportive supervision, the PM creates a positive and productive work environment for their team.

In 2017, a study was conducted in Mozambique's Niassa Province to assess the benefits of offering supportive supervision to health workers in government health facilities. Qualitative findings from this study on the 'Support, Train and Empower Managers' (STEM) initiative demonstrated that health workers perceived an improvement in their performance, which they attributed to the supportive supervision provided by their supervisors through the STEM project intervention. Additionally, there were reports of increased motivation among health workers. An unexpected but noteworthy outcome of the intervention was the increase in participation and voice among health workers in the facilities where the intervention was implemented, which the participants directly attributed to the supportive supervision they received.[2]

The PM holds the responsibility of overseeing the entire team. However, if the PM is managing a sizeable health project team, they will only provide supportive supervision to those who directly report to them. These are typically the senior members within the team that are accountable to the PM for all their project activities. They submit their monthly or quarterly reports directly to the PM. From these senior team members, the PM usually selects mid-level supervisors that possess supervisory skills. The PM ensures they receive proper training on supportive supervision. These mid-level supervisors in turn supervise the peripheral level team members.

Thus, the peripheral staff members report directly to their immediate managers, who then report to the PM. Although these peripheral staff members are still accountable to the PM, they do so through an intermediary (mid-level) manager or supervisor. In some projects with a large team, the PM may even need to have more than one layer of mid-level supervisors.

Early in my global health career, I was tasked with overseeing an immunization project in Bangladesh. The project involved managing 230 staff members across 16 districts in a large geographical area. I directly supervised 6 skilled medical officers, who were local doctors, as well as a few other supporting staff. These medical officers supervised project officers, who in turn supervised community health workers and volunteers placed in more peripheral locations.

To effectively carry out their role, supervisors require suitable resources, such as supervision checklists (which outline essential performance areas and targets) and recording forms to document their observations, recommendations, and follow-up actions. They should also have access to training materials and job aids to give OJT to their supervisees. These tools must be concise, precise, and user-friendly.

Supervisory visits to project sites

To provide effective supervision to the team members, the PM should plan regular project site visits to supervise those that report directly to them. These sites are the locations where project activities are carried out. It is vital for the PM to make site visits regularly to observe how their direct supervisees conduct their tasks. Image 5.1 shows the arrival of the PM at a project site for conducting supervision.

The mid-level supervisors in the team need to do this as well for their supervisees. All supervisors must schedule supervision visits and include them in their work plan. They should be well-informed and trained on project activities and the steps involved in on-site staff supervision. If necessary they should receive refresher training on supportive supervision.

Supervisors require transportation, drivers, fuel, and per diem for site visits. These items should be included in the project budget and made

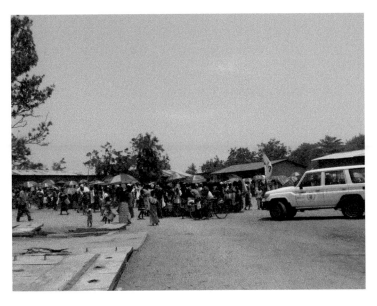

Image 5.1 Site visit in remote location for supervising food distribution by project staff in rural Burundi

available ahead of time. The location, time, and objectives of each visit should be well-planned.

Supervision should not always take place at nearby or easily accessible locations. Plans should include remote sites that did not perform well during previous supervision visits, as well as sites that routinely report high performance or where new activities have been introduced.

During site visits, it is important to observe staff and their activities. Not all project sites are active every day, and supervisory trips should be arranged for those sites where project activities will be taking place during the visit. Child vaccination may take place at selected sites on certain days of the week, to give an example. Thus, supervisory visits should be arranged for those sites (including mobile outreach units) where child vaccinations will take place and, on those days, when vaccination sessions have been planned. Supervisors should schedule sufficient time for site visits so that OJT can be provided to the supervisees if needed. The frequency of supervisory visits depends on various factors such as the need for OJT, problem-solving, supporting new sites or health centers, or encouraging newly recruited team members.

There are several activities that the supervisor needs to carry out during a site visit. These include collecting information through observation of site activities, listening to health workers and also the community members gathered at the sites for services or health education, reviewing records such as patient registers or pharmacy logbooks kept at the project sites, reviewing reports and recommendations from previous visits, and making a community visit to see how community members perceive the benefits they receive from the project and if they have any opinions or suggestions about these services.

The supervisor provides OJT to the site staff, if necessary, for instance, training a midwife on monitoring fetal heartbeat with a fetoscope. This usually includes several steps such as, demonstrating to the supervisee how a task is done; the supervisee practicing the specific skill; supervisor reviewing the practice session; and giving constructive feedback to the individual. If there are problems in carrying out a task, the supervisor helps the supervisee to find practical solutions to the problem. The supervisor gives feedback to the site staff, both positive and negative, and makes recommendations to the supervisee. The supervisor also jointly plans with the supervisee on following up on these recommendations.

At the end of a site visit, the supervisor uses the notes made during observations, OJT, and discussions to write a brief supervision report with the date and place of the visit. The supervisory checklist used during the visit is helpful for recording this information, particularly on how the staff has accomplished performance goals and targets. The written supervision report should include areas of success and accomplishments, concerns, any OJT given to the site staff, recommendations made to the supervisee during the visit, any plans for change, etc. These reports serve to determine if and how improvements are made and what still needs to be done at the site. Enhancing supervision reports with field photos is an excellent way to capture the features of a visit.

Spot checks

In the field of management, there is a phenomenon known as the 'Hawthorne effect,' where individuals tend to perform better when they know they are being observed.[3] To avoid this, supervisors sometimes conduct unannounced visits to project sites. During these visits, the supervisor prepares as they would for a regular visit but does not inform site staff of the exact day or time of the visit. Such surprise visits are often called *spot checks*.

The purpose of a spot check is to gain a realistic impression of how site staff conduct their activities when they do not expect to be supervised. However, some critics argue that this strategy can make individuals feel as though they are being suspected of wrongdoing, which can be demoralizing and goes against the spirit of supportive supervision. Ultimately, the decision to conduct spot checks will depend on various factors such as past supervisory reports, staff performance trends, and feedback from external sources such as a partner organization, government counterpart, or community representatives.

Staff performance appraisal

Besides supervisory visits to project sites, regularly reviewing the performance of project team members is indispensable. When done properly this review process contributes to supportive supervision. The appraisal process includes monitoring whether staff members are meeting their individual targets, and evaluating their performance in areas such as interpersonal relationships and professional growth. This process is known as *staff performance appraisal.*

By conducting these appraisals, supervisors ensure that all project employees are effectively working towards achieving project goals and objectives. It also helps supervisors establish more honest relationships with their supervisees and feel more confident in their supervisory roles. Team members gain a clear understanding of what is expected of them and how they are performing, which enhances their relationship with their supervisor.

Staff performance appraisal involves several key steps, which the PM and other supervisors should undertake with their supervisees in a sequential manner. While organizations may differ in their approach, we will discuss a simple system that many organizations have found beneficial.

Goal setting

At the beginning of the performance appraisal cycle, which typically lasts for one year, the PM meets with each individual team member that directly reports to them for initiating the appraisal process. Mid-level supervisors should do the same with their more peripherally placed supervisees. Thus, the *direct* supervisor of a staff member initiates the performance appraisal of that individual (supervisee).

The annual performance review cycle begins with the staff and the PM jointly deciding on the goals, objectives, or targets that the employee will achieve over the course of the review period. These are not the project's goals, objectives, or targets. They are personal and relate to the individuals in the project team. The question they should ask is: *What will I achieve during the performance review period (normally a year)?* This is best done during a meeting between the PM (supervisor) and the team member (supervisee), after the staff has had a chance to think through the goals and targets for the appraisal period.

It is important to ensure that these goals and targets are practical, and that they align with the health project's and organization's objectives. Before setting individual goals, it is helpful to review the project, department, and organizational goals. The team member's goals should contribute to the achievement of the strategic goals of the project and implementing organization.

A form is typically used to list the supervisee's goals or objectives and indicators or targets, along with any relevant notes, such as things that are deemed necessary for completing targets. This document is usually called the 'staff appraisal form' and provides a table with rows and columns for the objectives, targets, and spaces for scores or ratings for each row (objectives and targets). There is a column for brief comments as well. See Appendix C for a blank sample staff appraisal form.

Objectives and targets can be administrative, personal, or performance related. As examples, *administrative* objectives might include attending a certain percentage of team meetings, while *personal* development goals could involve reading technical books and presenting their key points at such team meetings. The *performance* or *technical* objectives, and targets can be as complex as ensuring medical supplies are ordered well in advance so that there is no shortage of essential medicines in the project warehouse during any quarter, or organizing a certain number of community health education sessions over the performance appraisal cycle. Or training a specific number of CHWs on the use of HIV rapid test kits for diagnosis of the disease.

Some organizations prefer performance and technical goal and objectives to be 'SMART.' The acronym stands for Specific, Measurable, Achievable, Relevant, and Time-bound. An example of a SMART objective for a PO might be "Teaching at least 20 CHWs in ten health centers how to prepare ORS in the first quarter of the year."

Breaking down annual targets into quarterly targets is ideal. For example, if a team member sets a goal to train 20 health center midwives on conducting normal delivery in a year, it is a good idea to divide this target number by quarters or months and list these smaller targets in the staff appraisal form. Such target breakdown allows the PM and their team member to review the performance quarterly or at six-month point to monitor the progress instead of waiting until the end of a full review cycle to make corrections and adjustments. Quarterly or semi-annual mini performance appraisal is discussed later in the chapter.

Establishing distinct goals or objectives and targets at the beginning of the appraisal period allows the project team member and the PM to clearly understand what the individual is supposed to accomplish. When everyone agrees on the objectives, it provides a shared understanding of what success looks like. Setting goals and achieving them can give team members a sense of satisfaction and lead them toward future career advancements.

Setting goals can also highlight areas where additional support or training may be needed. It is crucial for the PM to ensure that the objectives and targets are appropriate for each team member, and that they are not setting unrealistic expectations for themselves. In this way the PM can help protect the team from feeling overwhelmed or discouraged.

The staff appraisal form, whether in paper or electronic format, captures the objectives and targets agreed upon by the project team member and the PM. The PM then submits this document to the HR Unit/ Department of the Country or Regional Office at the start of the appraisal year.

Self-evaluation by staff

As the performance year comes to a close and it is time for doing appraisals of the team members, usually the HR Unit begins the formal staff performance review process. Each team member receives a copy of the document that was jointly developed with their supervisor at the beginning of the annual review cycle.

When they receive the staff appraisal form, the team member reflects on their own performance against the objectives and targets which they had agreed upon with their supervisor. They then provide their own evaluation of how well they performed. In Appendix C, the column under 'Ratings' has space for the staff to assess their own performance and give a self-assessment score that they feel is appropriate. This is done for each objective listed on the form.

For example, if the objective was to organize all eight community health education sessions and it was fully achieved, the staff member might give themselves a full score in that column. The scores usually range from 1 to 5, with higher scores indicating better performance in relation to the set objectives and targets. Lower scores indicate the opposite.

Some organizations use alphabet letters to indicate the ranking, as seen in the sample form in Appendix C. The supervisee tallies the self scores for each target and gives the total score at the end of the form. There is also a column (usually the rightmost column) where notes can be made. These notes can describe challenges that prevented the staff member from completing the target or list key reasons for a major success. The notes are usually short and relevant to the self-score. In this way, the team member completes the self-evaluation for all the goals and targets listed on the form, with appropriate notes. The supervisee then sends the document to the supervisor, who in this illustration is the PM and who directly supervises the staff whose performance is being reviewed.

Appraisal by supervisor

The PM then assesses the staff's performance based on their own observations and interactions with team members. The PM scores each objective and target set at the beginning of the cycle in a column next to the staff's self-assessment. These scores are then added to give the total score at the bottom of the form, right next to that given by the supervisee. They may also write notes in the rightmost column to explain their score for each area of performance. These notes serve to clarify any discrepancies between the staff's self-assessment and the PM's evaluation. In some organizations, HR requires the staff and PM to provide explanations in the notes column for very low or very high scores.

The PM then provides final notes in a designated space to explain the final score. In some cases, the appraisal form may include space for the PM to recommend salary increase, promotion, performance improvement, probation, or termination.

Joint performance evaluation session

After completing the written performance assessment, the PM and the supervisee will meet to discuss the scores and notes, that they used for evaluating the supervisee's tasks. See Image 5.2. This is an opportunity to ensure mutual understanding and agreement on staff performance and for the supervisor and supervisee to jointly review the scores and notes during the appraisal session.

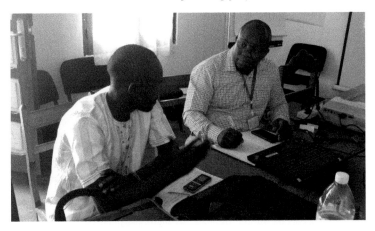

Image 5.2 Supervisor meeting with supervisee for performance evaluation in Central African Republic

The final scores may be altered based on this dialogue. It is important to strike an agreement on the scores and the notes. Following any adjustment and final scoring, the PM gives the document to the team member to provide any additional comments in a separate space in it. The team member then signs the document and returns it to the PM, either in paper form or electronically. The PM countersigns and submits the completed form to the HR Unit for record-keeping and further action. The signatures indicate the performance appraisal process has been completed.

In many organizations, the HR Unit will use this final document to determine staff salary increases or other financial incentives based on staff performance and the PM's recommendations. However, other organizations choose not to link salary increments to individual staff performance scores. Instead, each year they provide a certain level of increment across the board.

It is helpful for team members and supervisors to keep a copy of the staff performance document. This allows team members to refer to it periodically to improve their work output where necessary and provides supervisors with a reference for the following year's appraisal, as well as any needed feedback, support, and input.

Results of performance appraisal

After conducting a performance appraisal session with a supervisee, the PM may decide to recommend to the HR Unit a salary increase or promotion for the team member. However, if their work output and quality do not meet the acceptable level, the PM may need to put them on probation to closely monitor their performance and offer additional support.

Unfortunately, in some cases, there may be a need to terminate a team member, especially if they have not improved following poor previous appraisals or have violated rules and regulations. Also, there may be difficulties with interpersonal relationships involving the staff member. In such situations, it is crucial to follow the guidelines in the personnel policies and work closely with the HR Unit. Verbal and written warnings usually precede termination, and these should be documented, and the staff member should be informed of the decision to terminate at the appropriate time. Usually, the HR Unit takes the lead in terminating an employee and ensuring they return all assets belonging to the organization. All meetings, events, and exchanges involving the termination of the staff should be backed up with detailed notes. The PM shares these written records with the HR Unit.

The process discussed above for staff performance appraisal are the same for the PM as well as the mid-level supervisors in the project team who supervise the peripherally placed junior staff – their supervisees. The PM will need to ensure that everyone in the project team undergoes the annual staff appraisal. The PM is responsible for transmitting onward to the HR Unit the appraisal forms of all members of the project team.

Ongoing monitoring of staff performance

Performance appraisal meetings between supervisors and their supervisees are typically held once a year. However, it can be difficult for individuals to remember all the details of each team member's performance throughout the entire year when it is time for the annual appraisal meeting.

To address this challenge, a useful strategy for project team PMs and supervisors is to create confidential folders for each of their supervisees so they can keep track of all observations, reports, and performance-related events as these occur throughout the year. This way, at the time of the annual appraisal meeting, supervisors can share with their supervisees their notes on important goals, targets, and performance – both their strengths and weaknesses – that they documented throughout the year. This *ongoing monitoring* strategy allows for a more fair and practical performance review, based on documented facts over the entire appraisal period instead of doing a biased subjective appraisal.

Unfortunately, I have observed some PMs and supervisory staff hastily organizing performance appraisal meetings just before the appraisal submission deadline. In these cases, supervisors can only recall the incidents that come to mind at the time of the meeting, often focusing on negative or poor performances rather than recognizing the good things that team members have done throughout the performance period. This approach is unfair and can be demoralizing for team members. Therefore, utilizing the ongoing monitoring strategy is a more reasonable and effective way to conduct performance appraisals.

Mini performance appraisal

It is a useful practice for the PM not to wait for the time of annual performance appraisal but conduct appraisals at shorter intervals (e.g., quarterly or at mid-point) during the year. This type of performance review is similar to the annual process but is not done as elaborately as the annual one. The PM uses only a few key indicators in selected performance areas to do a rapid review of the supervisee's work. Thus, it can be done relatively quickly, informally, and every quarter or every six months. This shorter version of the appraisal is a *mini performance review*. This type of quick informal reviews over shorter intervals do not replace the annual performance review, which is more elaborate and formal involving the HR Unit.

The mini review offers several advantages.

- The PM and the staff members get the opportunity to communicate about work progress and performance more often.
- The PM can use this mini review as an occasion to identify early on whether the staff needs coaching or mentoring to perform project tasks. Where needed, the PM can address performance gaps and help correct the team members before problems become bigger.
- The annual appraisal scores from the PM do not come as a surprise or disappointment to the team member at the time of an annual review, since throughout the project cycle the progress or lack thereof has been discussed and addressed already at the mini review sessions.

The frequency of conducting mini reviews will depend on the number of team members the supervisors have, and the supervisees' level of experience. New or inexperienced staff members may need more frequent meetings with their PM and supervisors, while those with more experience may require less frequent reviews. If supervisors have too many supervisees, conducting frequent mini appraisals for each of them may be impractical.

The process for a mini review begins at the same time as the annual performance review process. The same HR form for the annual review is used for the mini review. The PM and mid-level supervisors jointly develop with their supervisees a set of performance goals for the annual review, which are then broken down into quarterly or mid-year goals. For instance, if a team member's annual goal is to conduct eight health education sessions throughout the year, a quarterly goal of two sessions can be set. At the end of each quarter, the mini review evaluates whether the team member organized the two sessions as planned. If there were issues, the supervisor can offer support and guidance to help them improve their performance in the following quarter.

During the mini review, the supervisor and supervisee score the goals and targets set for the quarter and note their progress and plans for improvement using the annual performance review form. This information informs the annual performance review at the end of the cycle. These mini reviews can help minimize the surprise and stress that often comes with annual performance reviews and instead, provide frequent feedback and support throughout the year. Such continuous feedback and support during the entire year can enhance the team members' learning, performance, and advancement in their careers.[4]

It is noteworthy that HR typically does not require documentation of mini reviews. These assessments are informal and intended mainly for the supervisors and their direct reports.

I have had the opportunity of working with an organization that had a structured system for supervisors to meet with their supervisees monthly. Together, they would establish a set of goals and targets for each quarter. Ahead of the monthly meeting, the supervisor would provide written feedback and suggestions to the supervisee related to the quarterly goals and targets. In turn, the supervisee would also provide written feedback and suggestions to their supervisor. During their one-on-one monthly meeting, both parties would elaborate on their written comments and create plans for future improvements. This meeting would be conducted online for approximately 30 minutes. This rewarding experience was valuable as it allowed both the supervisor and supervisee to meet more frequently and gain a better understanding of each other's expectations, performance progress, and need for support.

Supervising yourself

There is an adage that states, "*You cannot effectively lead others unless you can first effectively lead yourself.*" It is important for everyone in leadership roles to ensure they are growing professionally through self-supervision and self-discipline. When the time comes for you to lead a health project there are some key strategies that you can adopt for supervising yourself.[5]

- Monitor your work hours: If you are overworked you will need to find other activities outside of your work to help you relax and energize you. An exhausted PM is not an effective PM.

  > I will never forget what one colleague told me early on in my career when I was anxiously working extra hours in my office every day well into the evening: "*Long after you've had your heart attack and are gone, this organization will still be here.*" It is a memorable statement!

- Identify signs and symptoms of your own stress: Are you becoming increasingly irritated, fatigued, confused, frustrated, or dependent on tobacco or alcohol? Are you developing aches and pains? Are friends and colleagues trying to warn you? If the answer is "yes" to any of these, chances are you are stressed from work. You will need to relax and protect your physical and mental health.
- Avoid isolation and communicate with colleagues and loved ones: Working in isolation at your desk and hiding behind your computer only worsens loneliness, fatigue, and stress. Honest and reasonable communication with colleagues, friends, and family members helps to break isolation. Share with them how you feel at work and what you desire.
- Consult a mentor or advisor: They can help you with valuable guidance. Do not be afraid to reach out to them if you see in yourself the signals of overwork or stress.
- Recognize and celebrate every success: Even if no one else compliments you, praise yourself for your achievements. Do the same for others in your team to acknowledge them for their accomplishments.

Key takeaways

- For supervising team members, the PM needs to meet and interact with them for reviewing their performance.
- Supportive supervision is intended to help the project team do their work better and attain their goals and targets. It is the opposite of controlling or 'policing' individuals.
- The PM will need to ensure selected senior level staff members are trained and equipped so they can provide supportive supervision to peripherally placed team members as their supervisors.
- Besides other activities the supervisors have the responsibility to give OJT to their supervisees during project site visits.

- Spot checks can mitigate the 'Hawthorne effect.'
- Key elements of the annual staff performance appraisal process include goal setting, self-evaluation by staff, staff appraisal by supervisor, and organizing a joint performance evaluation session. This is followed by actions based on the results of the staff appraisal.
- Ongoing monitoring and mini performance reviews are useful strategies that can contribute to the annual staff appraisal process.
- You and the other supervisors in your team will benefit from self-supervision, which includes monitoring your own work hours, recognizing signs and symptoms of stress, avoiding isolation, consulting a mentor or advisor, and celebrating your successes.

Discussion questions

1. How can you ensure staff appraisal takes place for your teammates that are placed at distant project sites?
2. How is supportive supervision different from the more traditional controlling or 'policing' type of supervision?
3. Why is it beneficial to do a 'mini performance review' at shorter intervals during the appraisal cycle?
4. What are the pros and cons of conducting a spot check?
5. Multiple choice questions. Circle the number of the correct answer.
   5.1. The process of staff supervision involves:
       5.1.1. The PM regularly meeting and interacting with their team members.
       5.1.2. Team members reporting changes taking place in the community.
       5.1.3. The PM reporting to senior management on project accomplishments.
       5.1.4. The senior management developing job description for the PM.
   5.2. Supervisory visits to project sites require:
       5.2.1. Supervisors to find faults with their supervisees' project tasks.
       5.2.2. PMs to give health education to community leaders.
       5.2.3. Team members to write reports to the PM on the challenges the project faces.
       5.2.4. Supervisors to observe how their direct supervisees perform their project tasks.
   5.3. For staff performance appraisal the following sequence should be followed:
       5.3.1. Joint evaluation, self-evaluation by staff, goal setting, appraisal by supervisor.

5.3.2. Appraisal by supervisor, self-evaluation by staff, goal setting, joint evaluation.

5.3.3. Goal setting, self-evaluation by staff, appraisal by supervisor, joint evaluation.

5.3.4. Self-evaluation by staff, goal setting, joint evaluation, appraisal by supervisor.

5.4. A mini performance review of staff is characterized by:

5.4.1. Reducing the number of staff that are supervised.

5.4.2. Ongoing monitoring of staff performance.

5.4.3. Conducting an elaborate staff appraisal using all the indicators.

5.4.4. The use of the same HR form as in the annual review.

See correct answers on page 194.

Case study exercise

During the performance appraisal process, you come across the self-evaluation of one of your staff. Upon review, you notice that the individual has given themselves exceptionally high scores in almost all areas of performance. However, based on your analysis, this team member did not perform well enough to merit such high scores. Thus, you have chosen to provide your own more modest and appropriate scores.

As you prepare for the joint appraisal session with this supervisee, you wonder how to address this discrepancy in the scoring. How can you help your team member understand and accept your more realistic scores?

See Author's suggestion on page 197.

Notes

1 "Supervision," Scottish Social Services Council | Step into Leadership, accessed March 25, 2023, https://stepintoleadership.info/supervision.html

2 Madede, T., Sidat, M., McAuliffe, E. et al., "The impact of a supportive supervision intervention on health workers in Niassa, Mozambique: a cluster-controlled trial," *Human Resources for Health*. Last modified 2017, https://doi.org/10.1186/s12960-017-0213-4

3 Perera, A., "Hawthorne Effect: Definition, How it Works, And How to Avoid It," *Simply Psychology*, last modified February 8, 2023, www.simplypsychology.org/hawthorne-effect.html

4 "Performance Management: Traditional and Progressive Approaches," *Management Library*, last modified September 21, 2022, accessed April 11, 2023, https://management.org/performancemanagement/state-of-the-art.htm#anchor4292852898

5 "Why Self-Supervision is an Essential Skill?" Exforsys, last modified November 30, 2010, accessed April 19, 2023, www.exforsys.com/career-center/self-supervision/self-supervision-essential-skill.html

References

Exforsys. "Why Self-Supervision is an Essential Skill?" Last modified November 30, 2010. Accessed April 19, 2023. www.exforsys.com/career-center/self-supervision/self-supervision-essential-skill.html

Madede, T., Sidat, M., McAuliffe, E. et al. "The impact of a supportive supervision intervention on health workers in Niassa, Mozambique: a cluster-controlled trial." *Human Resources for Health*. Last modified 2017. https://doi.org/10.1186/s12960-017-0213-4

Management Library. "Performance Management: Traditional and Progressive Approaches." Last modified September 21, 2022. Accessed April 11, 2023. https://management.org/performancemanagement/state-of-the-art.htm#anchor4292852898

Scottish Social Services Council | Step into Leadership. "Supervision." Accessed March 25, 2023. https://stepintoleadership.info/supervision.html

Simply Psychology. 2023 "Hawthorne Effect: Definition, How it Works, And How to Avoid It." Last modified February 8. www.simplypsychology.org/hawthorne-effect.html

6 Communicating with project team members

In earlier chapters you have learned about building the health project team, developing detailed activity plans, improving team performance, and supervising project staff. In this chapter we discuss the team communication skills of the PM. As you assume the role of the PM for a global health project, effective communication with your team members becomes crucial throughout all project activities. Whether you are selecting and building your team, increasing capacity, supervising staff, managing the budget, or overseeing monitoring and evaluation, constant communication with your team is essential.

To excel as a PM, one must prioritize effective communication and foster positive interactions among team members. A positive and productive relationship between the PM and the team can lead to the success of a project. Thus, good communication practice is vital for project success.

Definition of communication

Webster's dictionary defines communication as *a process by which information is exchanged between individuals through a common system of symbols, signs, or behavior.* In the context of managing a global health project, team communication is the exchange of information within the team. It includes the PM's information exchange with their team members and communication between the team members themselves.

When every team member communicates clearly with one another, it eliminates misunderstandings, fosters a friendly environment, and helps everyone achieve work objectives efficiently and professionally. Unfortunately, poor communication is a significant issue in most workplaces today. According to a recent Gallup poll, only seven percent of U.S. workers strongly agree that communication is accurate, timely, and open where they work.[1] This and other similar statistics make it imperative that the PM and their health project team adopt a communication strategy that will encourage an open and efficient exchange of information.

DOI: 10.4324/9781003405245-7

Communication modes

For successful team communication, it is important to recognize there are four fundamental forms of communication, which include *verbal*, *written*, *visual*, and *non-verbal* methods. By effectively utilizing these four basic modes of communication, the PM and their teammates can improve collaboration and productivity.

Verbal communication

The most widely used form of communication is verbal communication, which is essential for promoting teamwork. Examples of verbal communication include face-to-face discussions, phone calls, and video conferencing, where people speak aloud and audibly. It is important to pay attention to the tone of voice used in meetings and to ensure that everyone speaks clearly and professionally.

When communicating verbally with the team, it is important for the PM to display confidence and seriousness. If team members detect uncertainty or lack of seriousness, they may disregard the PM's information or become skeptical. Using simple language in the verbal (and written) communications can reduce the risk of misunderstanding or wasting time clarifying. The PM should avoid repeating themselves, as this can cause the team members to lose interest in what is being said, and not take the PM seriously. The PM should simply state what they want the team to know or do, and if the teammates are clear about it, there is no need to repeat it. This also applies to written communication.

Written communication

Written communication within teams can take many forms, such as emails, letters, memos, texting, or even social media.

> Following the devastating Hurricane Dorian in 2019, our emergency health team in the Bahamas relied heavily on WhatsApp for most of our internal communications. Daily texting was necessary to exchange important information and stay in constant touch with the team. We didn't want to miss out on any urgent team meetings or not know to which health centers medical supplies would need to be delivered on a given day. The app allowed us to communicate effectively with each other as well as the external partners in the MOH.

However, written communication lacks the advantages of face-to-face dialogue. Facial expressions and body language are missing, making it more difficult to convey messages accurately. The reader's mood or circumstances may affect how they interpret an email or a text message for instance, potentially leading to a different impression than intended.

The PM needs to use clear and professional language, and ensure proper spelling, grammar, and punctuation are utilized when writing. Before sending any messages, they should review them carefully. They must keep written communications simple and concise, taking into account the needs and priorities of the recipients, who may communicate differently from the PM. This is especially important in cross-cultural settings, like those found in LMICs.

Visual communication

Visual communication involves the use of images in various mediums such as PowerPoint presentations, social media posts, diagrams, infographics, charts, and graphs. These visuals can relay a message on their own (e.g., infographics), along with written texts (e.g., images or charts), or visual aids (e.g., videos or PowerPoint slides) to illuminate and clarify a presentation or message. The PM should ensure that their team not only hears their message but can also see it clearly for better comprehension. When selecting design, color, and subject matter for the visuals, it is crucial to choose options that are easily visible and non-offensive to viewers. Additionally, it is important to consider the needs of individuals who may be visually impaired and to use large fonts and appropriate color contrast to accommodate their needs.

Non-verbal communication

During a conversation the PM's body posture, facial expressions, and hand gestures can convey powerful impressions to those around them. Positive signals, such as bright eyes, a smile, showing interest, and leaning forward while speaking, can readily connect the PM to the audience. In contrast, negative impressions can be created by slouching, fidgeting, avoiding eye contact, crossing the arms, or appearing disinterested when someone is speaking. It is critical to avoid these non-verbal signals, especially during in-person gatherings or video conferences where people can see each other.

Developing communication skills

Since effective communication is vital for a successful working relationship within the health project team it is beneficial to follow a set of guidelines for developing this skill.

Setting well-defined communication expectations

For preventing miscommunications and to help the team complete project tasks effectively it is necessary for the PM to set clear expectations for their team communications and also follow these rules themselves. Instructions must be precise and complete. This will help everyone understand when their tasks should be completed, when team meetings are scheduled, when progress reports are due, and when to make phone calls, and send emails among other things. By doing this, the PM will be able to anticipate when they will receive emails or phone calls from team members, when meetings will be held, and when they should expect responses and feedback. The team members will appreciate the organized approach to communication and are more likely to respond positively.

Intently listening to others

Most of us are familiar with the useful advice to "be a good listener." Stephen Covey said, "*Most people do not listen with the intent to understand; they listen with the intent to reply.*" It is important to try to understand the message the person is conveying and then respond in thoughtful ways. The wise PM is a good listener who genuinely listens with interest when someone speaks to them, even if it seems uninteresting.

People can tell when they are being heard versus when they are being ignored. During conversations with the team members, the PM should avoid giving off negative non-verbal cues such as a blank or bored look, fidgeting, turning away from the speaker, continuously looking at the computer screen, checking the clock or wristwatch, or walking towards the exit. These actions do not give them a good impression of one's ability to truly listen and focus on the matter at hand. By avoiding these negative cues, the PM can establish themselves as an active listener.

Arranging regular one-on-one meetings with team members

I have fond memories of a time when my supervisor at an organization set up weekly meetings with me. During these meetings, we both came prepared with notes and had a structured conversation about how my work week went. I would discuss my achievements, challenges, and situations that I faced, and together we would make plans for the following week. My supervisor provided feedback and advice, cautioning me when necessary and offering her support.

We would create a list of tasks for me to complete before our next meeting, and my supervisor would also make a list of things she would do to support me. I always looked forward to these meetings as these gave me the opportunity to have open and transparent conversations with my supervisor.

Regrettably, some managers in organizations view one-on-one meetings as a waste of time. They miss out on the chance to establish transparency and improve communication with their team members. The PM would do well to utilize these individual meetings for strengthening their working relationship with each teammate and gain insight into their tasks and challenges.

Taking notes during meetings and conversations

It is good practice to take notes during group meetings or one-on-one conversations with the team members. It is often difficult to remember everything that is discussed and decided upon during a conversation, and notes can help with recalling important details. Taking notes is also a key element of active listening.

To avoid slowing down conversations with notetaking, one might like to use digital tools such as cell phones or recording features on online platforms during meetings, which makes it easier to prepare and share notes with others.

Demonstrating a positive attitude in all types of communication

Maintaining a positive tone when project performance is going smoothly is easy. However, when the team makes a costly error, misses deadlines, or has differences of opinion, it can be challenging to keep one's cool. Sometimes, when things do not go as planned, people tend to withhold information because they fear that others may feel anxious or frustrated. However, it is important for the PM to communicate to the team any issues that may affect the project. Failure to do so can lead to anxiety, mistrust, and rumors within the team that cause morale to plummet and work quality to suffer.

A strong and positive leader remains calm and composed even in vexing situations. They control the temptation of becoming aggressive in communication when tensions mount. Experienced PMs plan ahead on how they will handle heated discussions. Instead of responding forcefully, using a professional and positive tone is much more effective in resolving difficulties. The teammates will respect the PM more, and they will not become dismayed or frustrated.

After every form of communication, whether it be verbal, written, over the phone, or through video conference, it is important to express gratitude to the listeners for their time and contributions, particularly during team meetings. This simple act of kindness will earn the PM the respect of their team members.

Ensuring communication is transparent and professional

To ensure clear communication among team members, it is best to use language that is easily understood by everyone. The PM should avoid using jargon and complex terms to make sure instructions and plans are easy to understand for everyone involved.

It is crucial for the team leader to be transparent in communication with the team and avoid withholding any relevant information from them. However, certain sensitive information should not be discussed during team meetings.

In some cases, it may be best to share information in stages, giving team members enough time to process it. Therefore, it is important to carefully choose the information to share, determine the amount of information to share, and decide when to share it.

Maintaining an open-door communication policy

Creating a friendly and approachable demeanor as a PM can foster better relationships with team members than appearing too busy, aloof, or difficult to reach. The PM ought to encourage open communication by establishing an open-door policy where team members can freely bring to the team leader suggestions and complaints, or seek their advice. It is important to actively engage with the team by walking around the office and visiting their workspaces to check on their progress or offer assistance. This approach can create a welcoming atmosphere that encourages good communication and strengthens relationships.[2] On the contrary, fear or distrust can hinder progress and damage relationships.

Requesting feedback from teammates and giving them feedback

Improving one's communication skills is possible by asking for feedback from team members. Creating a safe and open environment is essential where teammates feel comfortable sharing their thoughts on the PM's communication strategies and skills, as well as other issues. When receiving feedback, listening without interruption, being open-minded and avoiding being defensive are some vital skills that the PM should develop. They should take the time to reflect on the team's feedback and decide how it can be used to enhance their communication techniques. The PM should provide constructive feedback to their teammates on their communication strategies as well, since this can greatly improve team interactions.

Practicing public speaking

To effectively communicate with the team, the PM will need to project confidence, clarity, and a leadership tone. This means taking the time to organize one's thoughts, make notes, and thoughtfully deliver the comments, ideas, and instructions. While it may take some practice, it is worth the effort to avoid fumbling for words or rambling through the discussions.

> Early in my career I was terrified of public speaking. However, with practice, I overcame this fear. Well ahead of my presentation I would create brief speaker notes, rehearse my speech, practice my hand gestures, and track the time the presentation would take. I would go over the visuals such as posters and slides over and over again so my presentation would go smoothly. These steps helped me greatly and can help anyone wanting to improve public speaking.

Communication with remote or hybrid teams

When managing a team spread across a wide area, the PM would want to keep in mind that hybrid teams have become more common in recent years. Not all team members are in a central office, as remote work is becoming increasingly popular due to the emergence of difficult situations such as the COVID-19 pandemic, EVD outbreaks, and armed conflicts in many places. In some settings, the PM will manage their remotely located team with some or all of the team members coming together in person only occasionally for some special events, such as a retreat.

Emerging technologies for organizing virtual meetings have become essential in helping to bridge the distance between teammates. These days online platforms like Microsoft Teams, Skype, Webex, Zoom, and others are normal modes of communication for connecting with people working in different locations. Meetings and webinars can be held online with staff members and external participants located all over the world. It is interesting to see how even in remote villages of LMICs cell phones have become ubiquitous, and how so many people use them for conducting

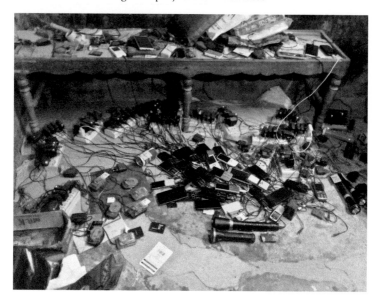

Image 6.1 Cell phone charging shop in Bangladesh
Credit: Mahfujur Rahman Nahid

daily business. Image 6.1, which shows how cell phones are being charged in a village market in Bangladesh, gives an idea of how popular the cell phone has become even in resource constraint rural areas.

There are a few best practices that a PM can consider for communicating with team members that work completely remotely or in a hybrid model. Let us look at these.

Selecting appropriate tools

Depending on the type of communication, the PM uses different communication tools and platforms. Tools such as email, chat, video conferencing, project management, and file-sharing software have become indispensable. The PM should select the tools that are reliable, secure, and user-friendly for everyone on the team. All team members should have access to the selected tools and know how to correctly use them.

To communicate more effectively and empathetically, the experienced PM uses multiple channels to connect with teammates. Different channels serve different purposes. For instance, emails are ideal for formal and detailed communication, chats are suitable for quick and informal information exchange, and video calls are useful for personal or team meetings.

Preparing well for virtual meetings

Time is wasted when individuals repeatedly try to access an online meeting when it has already begun but are unable to connect because they are not familiar with the software app or the login procedure. When organizing an online event, the PM ensures all participants have access to the same platform software on their devices and that they know how to use it. It is also a good idea to encourage participants to test their hardware and software before the event begins to ensure that they can connect without any issues. Conducting a test meeting prior to the actual event can be helpful in troubleshooting any technical difficulties and ensuring a smooth and successful online event.

Considering time zones and timely exchange of information

Not all team members or remote meeting attendees may be in the same time zone. This is particularly true if the meeting includes individuals from another country, such as a health program advisor based in an overseas regional office or the international headquarters of an NGO. If possible, the PM should consider recording the conference call on the online platform so that those who cannot attend live can still access the information later.

When different time zones are involved, one should prioritize timely communication to ensure that messages are sent and received promptly. Recipients must receive the information they need in a timely manner so that they can take appropriate action within the expected timeframe.

Setting up clear expectations

When communicating remotely, the PM establishes clear goals, responsibilities, frequency, format, and the appropriate content of communication for team members. Depending on the meeting needs, one may choose to have daily check-ins via chat especially for the direct reports, weekly video conferences for the team, or bi-weekly emails to share updates and feedback. Experienced PMs make sure to agree with their team on response times, level of detail, and tone of communication. It is essential to communicate these expectations clearly and regularly with the team and be willing to adjust them as needed.

Demonstrating respect and sensitivity

When communicating remotely, sometimes it can be easy to overlook the importance of being respectful and empathetic. Emails and chats can feel impersonal, especially when managing projects in LMICs where team members may come from different linguistic and cultural backgrounds. Furthermore, there may be differences in individual personalities. Having sensitivity, particularly towards team members with diverse backgrounds, is a valuable trait to possess. Showing respect and empathy towards each member can help build trust, rapport, and loyalty within the project team.

Using feedback to adjust and improve

As previously mentioned, receiving feedback is important. It is necessary to ask the team members for their candid feedback on their experiences, particularly with remote communications. The PM would want to provide them feedback as well. By exchanging feedback on the effectiveness of the channels utilized for remote communications, communication style, and the frequency and appropriateness of the communications, the PM is better equipped to adjust and improve remote team interactions.

Conducting project team meetings

When working on a project, a substantial amount of the PM's communication with team members occurs during team meetings. Planning these meetings carefully to ensure they are productive is essential. Typically, the PM leads the discussions and encourages participation from all team members. The PM also records the meeting's outcomes or assigns someone to take notes for follow up on any decisions or actions agreed upon during the meeting.

Preparation for team meetings

Purpose and objective

When planning team meetings, the PM has a clear purpose and objective in mind. Their team members are informed of the reason for gathering, so they understand the value of the meeting. Without a clear purpose, team members may feel their time is being wasted, leading to resentment towards meetings.

Balanced duration for meetings

To ensure engagement, team meetings are usually planned for no more than 90 minutes. Meetings that are too long can lead to boredom and disinterest, with team members switching off and thinking about their tasks they must get done. However, meetings that are too short may not cover all the necessary topics. Finding a balanced duration for meetings is key, ensuring participants see the value in attending.

Clear outcomes

Besides the purpose, there must be clarity on the *outcome* of the team meetings. PMs decide what would they and the team want to get out of the meeting. For example, one could have a planning meeting to generate new ideas for a project activity, such as building a new rural health post. Again, a meeting could be organized to determine the steps needed to tackle a problem faced by the project, like developing protocols for staff during a disease outbreak, such as the recent COVID-19 pandemic. Celebrating a project achievement sometimes can also be a valid purpose of team meetings, such as congratulating the team for reaching the polio vaccination targets ahead of schedule.

Adequate communication

It is better to communicate more than less when working on a project. If someone is unsure whether to communicate with the team members frequently or infrequently, it is best to communicate more often. The project team members, particularly those who work remotely, may feel the need to consult with the PM regularly. They want to keep the PM updated on their progress and discuss any challenges they might be facing. If the PM lacks interest or does not provide support, the teammates may become demotivated, which can negatively impact their performance.

However, needless or excessive communication and too many meetings can also hinder one's work. This is especially true if the communication is only to demand progress reports or point out mistakes. A considerate PM strives to find the right balance and frequency of communication that works best for everyone in the team.

Number of participants

When planning a meeting, the PM carefully considers the number of attendees. A meeting with too many people can be difficult to manage and may not be as productive. Large meetings can be useful for sharing information and gathering opinions, but these may not be the best choice for discussing problems, reviewing policies, or making important decisions. For those types of discussions, it is more useful to have a smaller task force or committee meetings.

Meeting agenda

To make sure the meeting is successful, creating an agenda and sharing it with all participants ahead of time is essential. The PM prioritizes topics and allows enough time for discussions, questions, and comments, while still ending the meeting on schedule. Along with the agenda, they share relevant materials ahead of time that will be discussed during the meeting, such as a new prevention policy for disease outbreaks like COVID-19. By reviewing these materials ahead of time, participants can come prepared and ready to contribute to the discussion.

When creating a formal agenda for a meeting, the PM includes the name of the meeting (such as "Monthly Project Team Meeting"), the date, time, and location of the meeting, and the purpose of the meeting (such as "re-organizing project activities to respond to a health emergency"). The agenda should then list the discussion topics that will be covered during the meeting, along with the amount of time allocated for each topic and the names of those who might lead the discussions. Additionally, there should be a section for "Any Other Business" (AOB), where participants can suggest any additional topics for discussion that are not on the agenda.

In the event of an unforeseen crisis situation, calling an emergency meeting may become necessary. In such cases, creating and circulating an agenda may not be feasible. However, for regular meetings, an agenda is necessary to ensure participants are prepared to actively take part in the discussions.

Seating arrangement

For large group meetings, a circle or a semi-circle seating arrangement is ideal. This gives the best chance for individuals to see each other, make eye contact, and observe and use body language. For meeting with individuals, face-to-face seating is ideal.

Backup plan

One should be prepared for equipment failure during meetings. Technical issues can cause unnecessary delays and disruptions. To avoid this, it is helpful to have a backup plan in place. This could include having a technician available to fix a technical problem, or arranging a backup microphone or projector in case the one the presenter is using unexpectedly quits during the presentation. Additionally, power outages are common in many areas, and having a generator or battery backup for equipment is important. Printing out materials ahead of time to be circulated in the event of slide projection failure is a smart idea. Lastly, the PM should have alternative plans for discussions or exercises during team meetings, should there be a technical failure lending extra time at hand.

Types of meetings

There are several types of meetings to organize. At times the PM may need to share information that affects their team members and their work on the health project. Staff education and policy development meetings are held on occasion. At other times there may arise a need to make joint decisions, solve problems, or simply have fun activities to build up the project team.

Status update meeting

One of the most common types of meetings the PM leads is the routinely held project status update meeting. These meetings usually occur weekly, or bi-weekly, and all teammates should know the time and location. Most often, there are updates from team members on their activities and sharing of plans for upcoming tasks. Using the DAP for this purpose is an excellent idea. Status update meetings help keep everyone informed and motivated.

> When I managed the global health project in Nagorno Karabakh, I had sub-teams within my larger project team, each sub-team working on specific tasks. During weekly team meetings, each sub-team reported on their work progress. I could see how this strategy gave our project team a chance to support each other, offer advice, and help when needed. For example, when one sub-team was struggling to organize medications in our pharmaceutical warehouse due to staff shortage, another sub-team stepped in to help with the work. These meetings fostered healthy competition, mutual interest, and valuable support, building camaraderie among our team members. It was a rewarding experience for the entire team.

Information dissemination meeting

Often the PM or someone else in the team or from outside the project team shares important information that the team members need to know and act upon. These are information dissemination meetings. The meeting participants may ask questions for clarification but not get into discussions or debates. For instance, an HR department colleague from the country or regional office may provide the latest information on how the staff needs to fill out the recently re-designed timesheets. The decision to use this new type of timesheet throughout the organization has already been made and is not up for discussion or modification. The meeting is solely for giving information and orientation on the new timesheet.

As participants are only receiving information and not necessarily interacting with the speaker or with each other, these types of meetings tend to become uninteresting. To prevent fatigue, the PM can plan short breaks between sessions at perhaps 90-minute intervals or sooner. The presenter can make the long presentations of complex topics more interesting and engaging so the contents are not dry, but easy to understand. The use of multiple formats such as presentations, video clips, skits, simulations, and small group exercises, can keep everyone engaged and avoid monotony or lethargy.

Planning meeting

The PM organizes planning meetings which ideally should be quite participatory with everyone making contributions to the implementation plans for project activities. For example, if the PM wants to extend the health project to a neighboring district the team members should participate fully and provide their inputs on how to achieve this. At the planning meeting the team might jointly identify additional resources that will be required such as medicines, transport, and training materials, as well as anticipate any potential problems, and develop plans to monitor the progress of the project tasks. The new plan for extension will include details about the activities, deadlines, points of contact, and progress monitoring scheme.

> During technical workshops in many countries, I have led health strategy planning meetings with local health project teams. These meetings involved presentations, discussions, small and large group exercises, and role-plays. The local teams actively participated with high enthusiasm and developed detailed strategies for health programming in their countries. See Images 6.2 and 6.3 for examples from Sierra Leone and Burundi.

Problem solving meeting

During problem-solving meetings, the PM or a team member brings up a challenge that needs attention. These challenges could be related to internal policies, external factors that affect the project or team, or difficulties that the health project is facing. The first step is to clearly define the problem, supported by information and evidence. Then, team members who are directly involved with the issue work together to find a solution, with guidance from the PM. This approach encourages team members to take ownership of the practical solutions they generate.

To ensure that all participants in problem-solving and planning meetings understand the key points discussed, it is important to write down

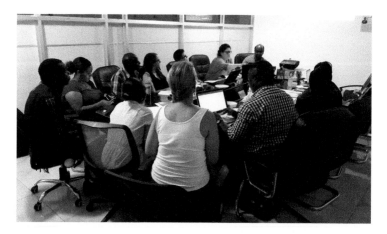

Image 6.2 Planning meeting with health project team in Sierra Leone

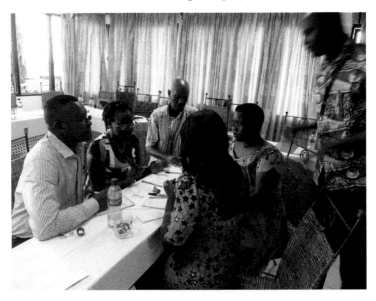

Image 6.3 Small group activity as part of a planning workshop in Burundi

all the key action points. This includes the tasks and sub-tasks that each team member is expected to carry out. Sharing these action points within the team is crucial. PMs follow up with individuals to ensure that specific tasks that were agreed upon are being completed.

Team building meeting

Many organizations and projects promote the idea of gathering staff in one place where colleagues can relax and have fun. These events can be referred to by different names, but we will call them 'team building meetings.' Bringing teammates together for games and other enjoyable activities helps foster collaboration through informal interactions. Such meetings can boost team morale and productivity.

> I had a remarkable experience with a team building initiative while working with an organization. Every Friday afternoon, just before the end of the workday, the entire organization's staff in the office would gather in a large conference room for a couple of hours of refreshments, music, games, skits, and other fun activities. We called this the 'Happy Hour.' Sometimes, these events were organized to observe special occasions such as national holidays, sports events, cultural celebrations, and more. With costumes, decorations, games,

and skits, these events turned into festivities. The organization allocated funds for these gatherings, and there was even a competition among staff to organize the most enjoyable Happy Hour. The laughter, food, and fun helped bring people together, creating strong bonds among staff and leading to the building of an effective team.

Team members appreciate and respond well if they know ahead of time the purpose of the upcoming meeting. This allows them to prepare and be aware of whether it will involve sharing information, making plans, solving problems, or engaging in team-building activities. Such preparation helps team members to respond positively and effectively during the meeting.

Managing team meetings

It is the PM's responsibility to manage the flow of discussion, meeting time, and interpersonal differences during team meetings. When a discussion tends to become stagnant or uninteresting, raising questions or introducing new items for discussion helps keep the flow going. Starting and ending meetings on time without allowing the discussion to go beyond the allocated time, and ensuring civility among the participants even when there may be dissent and disagreements, are critical features of managing meetings effectively.

A successful PM encourages team members to freely share and explain their views at group meetings and in personal communications without the fear of being reprimanded. They promote the expression of ideas and suggestions, even if they initially seem impractical or far-fetched. This approach allows the team to share and consider innovative concepts during the meeting, which can enrich the health project.

During meetings, a few people sometimes tend to dominate the conversation and not give others a chance to speak. These individuals are usually outspoken and influential in society and the project team, which leads them to behave in a dominating way. Unfortunately, this can be frustrating for others who want to share their thoughts and contribute to the conversation but feel subdued. Allowing this behavior to continue can make the 'quieter' individuals feel left out and unimportant, and it can create the impression that the PM only listens to a few vocal team members.

By discussing this behavior with the vocal teammates privately and asking them to allow others to speak so they too can share their thoughts during meetings the PM can address this issue. It is possible that these vocal team members have great ideas and potential for leadership, but just need guidance on how to share their ideas without overwhelming the rest of the team during meetings. The PM's role is to support the team and help everyone work together effectively.

If on the other hand, the PM notices some team members always remain quiet, it may be helpful to approach them directly during team meetings and invite them to share their thoughts and ideas. This lets them know that their contributions are valued.

Key takeaways

- A PM always needs to communicate with their team members. Thus, they need to become an effective communicator with good communication skills.
- There are four main modes of communication: verbal, written, visual, and non-verbal.
- Everyone including the PM should speak clearly and professionally paying attention to the tone of voice in all verbal communications.
- Written communication is relatively difficult as the advantage of face-to-face dialogue, facial expressions, and body gestures is missing.
- Visual communication allows the audience to *see* one's message for better understanding.
- Setting clear communication expectations will allow a structured approach to communication. Team members appreciate this and respond positively.
- Listening to others with genuine interest even if the subject is uninteresting is an important communication skill. This helps team members to put their trust in the PM.
- Having regular one-on-one meetings with team members and using these to build a stronger relationship with them is a good practice on the part of the PM.
- Taking notes, demonstrating a positive attitude in all communication, ensuring communication is transparent and professional, and maintaining an open-door communication policy are some of the important traits of a successful communicator.
- Requesting feedback from teammates and giving them constructive feedback is important for PMs.
- Virtual meetings have become increasingly popular and important in recent years. The PM and project team members at distant project sites routinely connect through online platforms.
- All participants should test their hardware and software before starting an online meeting.
- Considering time zones and timely exchange of information is important.
- There must be clarity on the purpose and the outcome of team meetings.
- An agenda is important to circulate among all participants before a meeting.
- For meetings, especially when equipment is used, one must always have a backup plan.

- Team building meetings bring the teammates together to have fun and games. These informal interactions contribute greatly to building better collaboration and team spirit.
- The PM is responsible for managing the flow of discussion, meeting time, and interpersonal differences during team meetings.
- A PM with good communication skills encourages active participation from all team members in planning and problem-solving meetings.

Discussion questions

1. What are the different types of project meetings? Which one does not require active contribution or discussion from the participants?
2. When team members work at distant project sites how can a PM communicate with them routinely? Which communication tools will you prefer to use? How frequently?
3. What are the different modes of team communication? What are the advantages and disadvantages of each one?
4. Table 6.1 contains seven numbered items covered in this chapter, with short descriptions in the right column. However, these descriptions are not arranged in the correct order and do not match the items on the left. Match each numbered item to its description on the right and correctly write the corresponding letter of the description in the middle column.

Table 6.1 Multiple choice questions

Match the following with the answers in the last column	Insert letter of the correct answer	Answer
1. Remote communications		A. Are perhaps the most common form of communication.
2. Planning meetings		B. Requires confidence, clarity, and leadership tone. These can be improved with practice.
3. Written communications		C. Are arranged for having fun, food, games, etc.
4. One-on-one meetings		D. Involve active participation of team members.
5. Team building meetings		E. Necessary for team members that do not work in one location all the time.
6. Verbal communications		F. Are difficult in the absence of dialogue, facial expressions, and body gestures.
7. Public speaking for a PM		G. Are seen by some as timewasters.

See correct answers on page 194.

Case study exercise

Imagine you have been recently promoted to a higher position in your organization. Congratulations! In your previous role, you were responsible for managing a peri-urban global health project on the outskirts of Mumbai, India. The project has a staff of 135 members, ten of whom you had directly supervised in the office and the others had been based in distant project sites, coming to the office only on certain days of the month and returning to project sites to work there for the rest of the month.

Your replacement, Vinod, has been appointed as the new PM and you are providing him with a detailed handover of the project for a few days before transitioning into your new role. You have noticed that Vinod is a good listener and takes notes during your meetings, but he does not seem to have experience in remote or hybrid communications.

To ensure Vinod is successful in connecting regularly with all 135 team members, what advice can you give him?

See Author's suggestion on page 197–198.

Notes

1 Jennifer Robison, "Communicate Better with Employees, Regardless of Where They Work," Gallup Workplace, Gallup, Inc., June 28, 2021, www.gallup.com/workplace/351644/communicate-better-employees-regardless-work.aspx
2 Cliff Goodwin and Daniel B. Griffith, *Supervisor's Survival Kit* (Columbus, Ohio: Pearson Prentice Hall, 2006), 76.

References

Goodwin, Cliff and Griffith, Daniel B. *Supervisor's Survival Kit*. Columbus, Ohio: Pearson Prentice Hall, 2006.
Robison, Jennifer. "Communicate Better with Employees, Regardless of Where They Work." Gallup Workplace. Gallup, Inc. June 28, 2021. www.gallup.com/workplace/351644/communicate-better-employees-regardless-work.aspx

7 Interacting with external stakeholders

In the previous chapter, you learned about how the PM and the health project team communicate with each other. In this chapter you will see that it is vital for a PM to also establish and maintain positive relationships with various *external* stakeholders. These stakeholders include local communities, government offices (especially those under the MOH), and donor agencies supporting the health project. The PM may also need to build relationships with private sector companies, private medical providers, journalists, UN organizations, and external visitors.

This chapter will focus on how the PM and project team interact with major external stakeholders who have an interest in the project and can affect or be affected by its outcome. In this chapter, we explore the dynamics of these relationships.

Major external stakeholders

The list of external stakeholders below is not exhaustive, but here is a discussion of the key ones that are important for a global health project operating in an LMIC.

Community leaders and members

Within most villages, urban, and peri-urban areas, there are typically local organizations made up of community leaders and members. In an LMIC village, for example, there may be a village development committee (VDC) and a village health committee (VHC). In addition to these formal groups, there are often village chiefs and elders who hold significant influence in their communities where the health project may be operating. In peri-urban settings, similar committees may be referred to as community development committees (CDCs) and community health committees (CHCs).

DOI: 10.4324/9781003405245-8

Ideally, these committees plan and execute activities that benefit their community members. The committee leaders and members meet regularly, keep records of their decisions and plans, monitor progress, and address any issues that arise. They may also maintain fund accounts that community members contribute to. Committees may lobby local authorities for things that would benefit their communities. Active committees carry out these tasks for the betterment of their community. In many places though, some committees that were originally formed with good intentions may no longer exist after some time has elapsed due to various reasons, or they may exist but are not very active.

Religious leaders

The PM could be managing a global health project in an area where religious leaders actively preach, teach, counsel, and help community members in spiritual and material ways. They can be extremely influential among their followers. Despite their primary responsibility and passion being spiritual work, these religious leaders are often very willing to serve their communities with health needs. They minister at religious places of worship, such as churches, mosques, and temples, which are often large gathering places where communities can access health messages and services.

The MOH

If one works for an NGO that supports the MOH, then the MOH is considered an external stakeholder for the project. On the other hand, if the PM is part of the MOH managing a health project, then the NGOs that support the MOH project are the external stakeholders. There is a collaborative relationship between the MOH and the NGOs, each supporting the other. This book primarily discusses the management of international or local NGO health projects.

The health ministry has multiple programs and offices, for example, the Nutrition Program, Expanded Program on Immunization (EPI), and Family Planning Program. Each program normally has its own office and staffing structure within the MOH.

The MOH provides government health services at several administrative levels of a country:

National or central level

At this level, nationwide health policies, plans, budgets, and coordination with non-governmental and governmental organizations, as well as international donor agencies are established for the healthcare of the country's population. Teaching and referral health institutions are mainly located in the country's capital or large cities, and they often serve as tertiary level hospitals.

The central level of the MOH operates national pharmaceutical warehouses, which distribute medicines and supplies country-wide through an elaborate supply chain management system. It provides training for doctors, nurses, and technicians in allied fields through government institutions established at national, regional, and district levels. Government health research institutes, post-graduate medical schools and hospitals, and medical institutions specializing in certain areas (e.g., heart diseases) also function at the national and regional levels.

In times of emergency, such as the COVID-19 pandemic or a hurricane, the MOH offices at the national level coordinate emergency response initiatives in collaboration with the lower levels.

State, provincial, or regional level

In this next level, the MOH administration, hospitals, and pharmacy warehouses are responsible for implementing the national MOH health policy and managing the health budget allocated for their state or province. Typically, the regional offices, hospitals and warehouses of this secondary level are situated in the state/provincial capital or a major city within the state, province, or region.

District level

Government healthcare services are available in the district communities through a network of hospitals, health centers, and district pharmacies. The district MOH office oversees all healthcare functions including medical and pharmaceutical services, logistics, training, and budgets.

Sub-district or local level

There are relatively small primary healthcare service centers, health posts, and dispensaries that serve communities in villages, urban and peri-urban areas. Ideally, patients receive basic health services at these primary healthcare centers in their local communities. If there are complications, patients are referred to the district level. For instance, the midwife at a primary healthcare center or health post can usually conduct a normal delivery in most LMICs. However, maternity patients with complications such as a breech presentation or hand prolapse will be referred to the next higher level, which is the district hospital.

Other non-health government ministries

Besides the MOH there are other ministries, with which the PM may need to interact while implementing the global health project. These could be the Ministries of Education, Agriculture, Religious Affairs, and others. These non-health ministries at the local, provincial, or national level may impact the health project in many ways.

Non-government voluntary agencies

In the same location where the health project operates, one may encounter various voluntary agencies involved in community development work. These agencies are similar to your NGO that is implementing the health project, in that they too are not affiliated with the government and are therefore referred to as 'non-government' organizations.

International and national NGOs

There are various types of NGOs, including international agencies, regional or local organizations. These organizations may focus on health-related activities or non-health programs such as small farming, fisheries, microcredit, income generation for women, disaster relief, or education for children. All NGOs operating in LMICs must follow national laws and government policies and guidelines when implementing their health and non-health projects. The PM is aware of the services provided by NGOs active in the project location, and they establish collaborative relationships with them to enhance their health project's success.

Besides these standalone NGOs there are coalitions of NGOs that join together to operate large initiatives in LMICs. These increasingly popular coalition projects involve like-minded NGOs forming an alliance to apply for donor funding. Although not all partnering organizations may be focused on health programming, each brings its strengths and specialties to the coalition, using donor funds to benefit the project communities. These are typically large-scale, comprehensive projects that span extensive areas of an LMIC. The PM or 'Chief of Party' of a coalition project collaborates with all other organizations' project leads and team members working in the coalition to ensure the project's success.

Community based organizations

In many communities, there are indigenous organizations that operate at the grassroots level within the community. These organizations may be connected to government ministries and help to implement their programs within the community as contractors. For example, if a government program installs hand pumps for water, it may engage a community-based organization (CBO) to perform the work. In some cases, CBOs operate under the government's authority as its extension, with their staff being government employees.

Alternatively, a CBO may be independent of the government but still supports government policies and facilitates program operations within the community. These non-government CBOs operate with their own staff and volunteers without government influence. They may work on health projects or non-health projects in their communities, such as securing low-interest loans from local banks to fund income-generating projects for women or supporting farmers with seeds and tools to meet their agricultural needs.

Faith based organizations

Religious or faith-based organizations (FBOs) are often active in communities, providing benefits to community members. Both international and local FBOs serve communities operating on the basis of their religious beliefs and convictions.

FBOs often run private hospitals and health centers in many countries, and in some locations, they also operate nursing schools and institutes for medical technicians. These health facilities are generally well-supported and staffed, and the communities they serve readily recognize their contributions. In the geographical areas where the PM is leading a global health project, there may be an FBO hospital, health center, or a mobile outreach health post operating where community members receive health services. Partnering with these FBOs and their facilities can be advantageous for the health project.

United Nations and humanitarian organizations

There are several UN organizations that are not grouped under any other category mentioned here. These include WHO, UNICEF, UNDP, WFP, UNHCR and others, which may be operational in or around your global health project location. Some of these organizations support development programs, such as UNDP and UNICEF, while others like the UNHCR are focused solely on humanitarian crises. Meanwhile, there are those that work in both contexts, such as WHO, UNICEF, and WFP.

Additionally, there are international organizations such as ICRC, IFRC, and MSF (also named Doctors Without Borders) that work in disasters and humanitarian conflict situations. For example, IFRC works in natural disaster contexts, while ICRC's mandate is to work in conflict situations. And MSF works in both.

Funding agencies

If the PM is managing a government or NGO project that has received funding from donor organizations, it is likely that the donor agencies have a main office at the national level in the capital city of the LMIC where the health project operates. Sometimes, they may only have an office in a neighboring country or maintain a regional office overseeing multiple LMICs, including the country of your project operation. The donor organization that invested in the health project is interested in the project's success and is willing to support the PM and their project team as they implement the project.

In certain situations, several donor agencies join together to fund a project, especially if it is a large initiative with many interventions or if it is a multi-year project. Each donor agency may commit to funding specific interventions or providing funding for specific geographical locations of the health project. In such a 'pooled fund' mechanism, there is usually one agency that leads the consortium of donors. The PM's interactions with the consortium in relation to the health project take place mainly through this lead donor agency.

Private sector practitioners and facilities

In this context, private sector practitioners are the individuals, agencies, and health facilities that are not part of the government medical system under the MOH. Usually these belong to the for-profit commercial sector. In many resource-constrained communities, such as rural and semi-urban areas, traditional health service providers play key roles in healthcare. These providers are the traditional and religious healers, village doctors and pharmacists, and traditional birth attendants. Being mostly untrained in modern health care, they often resort to incorrect medical practices. However, community members in LMICs often prefer to visit these local traditional providers instead of receiving treatment from trained physicians at recognized health centers.

Some government doctors and midwives establish their own private practice in the communities they serve, sometimes making it difficult to distinguish between the government and private systems. Private sector facilities, such as those set up by non-government agencies like FBOs, CBOs, or local and international charity organizations, can range from small health centers to large hospitals located in peripheral or central towns. Private practitioners and health facilities often fill critical gaps that may exist in the government sector.

When managing a global health project in a community, the PM may encounter private sector practitioners and medical establishments that can impact the health project.

Financial institutions

Financial institutions such as government or privatized banks and credit unions may be present in the project areas. These establishments are commonly used by members of the project communities for their banking needs. Sometimes, these entities offer bank loans to eligible community members. The PM needs to understand the loan and funding mechanisms offered by these local financial institutions, since these can benefit those the project is trying to help in the communities.

Collaboration with external stakeholders

An effective PM builds and nurtures relationships with as many external stakeholders as possible. The main goal of this collaboration is to create mutual benefits for both the health project and the external stakeholders. This book specifically focuses on collaboration of PMs managing global health projects for international or national NGOs. Therefore, the MOH and all other government and non-government entities mentioned above are considered external stakeholders for the PM and the NGO implementing the health project.

Community leaders and members

To effectively engage with the communities where the health project operates, it is necessary for the PM or project team members to regularly organize meetings with community leaders and members. One example is a public meeting held on the project site to inform villagers about a new health project or intervention, such as distributing malaria bed nets or providing de-worming activities for children. These meetings also provide an opportunity to gather feedback and ideas from the community.

Smaller meetings can be held with community leaders to discuss health issues and project activities aimed at addressing these issues. These meetings are also useful for solving difficulties with project operations. Group meetings may also be organized for patient groups or mothers' groups to provide health education.

PMs establish good relationships with influential community leaders who can help facilitate project activities and solve problems in their communities. These leaders are often part of VDCs and VHCs, which are made up of community members. These committees, in particular the VHCs can be valuable partners for the health project, providing support and advice to the project team members. If these committees have not been active for some time, it may be necessary for the project team to revive them.

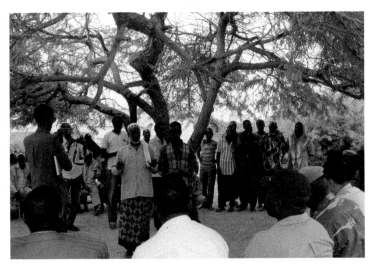

Image 7.1 Meeting with community members in the Democratic Republic of the Congo

Interacting with community leaders and members as seen in Image 7.1 is essential for a successful health project. The PM follows these steps to engage effectively with them:

- They arrange both informal and formal meetings with community leaders to discuss the establishment of a functional VHC (and/or VDC) in the village. The PM inquires about any previous committees and why they are no longer effective. They then work with leaders to activate the committee or establish a new one, which may take some time and patience.
- The PM explains the health project and its benefits to villagers in simple terms, while seeking agreement of community leaders on project goals. In the event of disagreement, one questions about past misunderstandings or disappointments with similar health projects and seeks advice from community leaders. Unfortunately, there may have been times when it appears some PMs and team members failed to treat community leaders and members with respect. Perhaps this happens because they perceive themselves to have a higher social and financial status relative to the villagers. However, one must keep in mind, everyone deserves respect regardless of their position in life. U Thant, the third secretary general of the United Nations had aptly said, *"Every human being, of whatever origin, of whatever station, deserves respect. We must each respect others even as we respect ourselves."* Wise PMs give these community leaders and members genuine respect to gain their trust and secure support for the project.

- Once a functional VHC is established, the PM schedules regular discussions and events with committee members to share information, solve problems, try new ideas, and review health progress in the community. They ensure meetings are interesting and engaging with two-way conversations between committee members and the project team, using these discussions for learning and teaching.

> One time on a monitoring visit to South Sudan, I learned from a discussion with a VHC why the village women were reluctant to come to the small delivery unit that the local health project had constructed adjacent to the rural health center. This modest delivery unit had a wooden delivery table equipped with stirrups, special adjustable lamps, disposable sheets, instruments, medicines, and more. Additionally, the project hired and trained a local midwife to perform normal deliveries at this unit. I found the delivery unit well-organized and spotlessly clean. And yet, most of the deliveries in this community continued to take place in the village huts in unhygienic conditions, with untrained birth attendants. This led to a high number of maternal and newborn deaths in this area.
>
> At this gathering the VHC leaders and members explained to me and the project team members that came with me that the village women preferred to give birth on the floor in a squatting position. They were not comfortable climbing onto a high table and having their feet placed on stirrups! This was a very important learning for me and my colleagues from the project.
>
> During our conversation with the VHC, we discussed a possible improvement for the project's delivery unit. We came to the decision that hiring a carpenter to saw off the legs of the wooden table to lower it to the floor level would be a good thing. This adjustment would still ensure that safe deliveries are conducted in a clean and hygienic environment. The VHC members expressed satisfaction with this decision and gladly offered to share the news of this change with their community. They agreed to inform community members about the importance of coming to this delivery unit for childbirth instead of delivering babies in their huts.
>
> The VHC and health project colleagues had a valuable experience of learning and teaching involving each other. By sharing ideas and collaborating to make changes, everyone benefited.

- Global health projects can benefit from the assistance of VHCs that help select motivated individuals from the community to serve as volunteers or village health workers. These committees keep an eye on the work of these grassroots-level workers and volunteers, encourage and support them in their work, and provide valuable feedback to the project team.

- VHCs also organize community gatherings to educate local residents on health-related topics, distribute materials like malaria bed nets and health supplies such as ORS packets. They encourage community members to participate in these events, provide meeting venues, and follow up on project tasks. This support helps to improve health projects and their impact on the community.
- Additionally, VHCs often partner with projects to bring vital clinical services to their community. They take ownership of these project activities with their guiding, monitoring, and problem-solving roles.

> During my travels, I came across two inspiring examples of community-led health initiatives. In a small island community in the Philippines, a VHC played a significant role in supporting a health project. The VHC collaborated with local jeepney owners and drivers to transport pregnant women to the nearby hospital for delivery. When a woman went into labor, a VHC member would receive a call and contact a jeepney driver to quickly transport the patient. The health project would reimburse the driver for their service. The VHC successfully handled several complicated delivery cases each year, saving many lives in the process.
>
> Again, in a peri-urban community outside Mumbai, India, the CDC took charge of organizing and supervising health-related activities. The committee set up daily clinics with a trained medical doctor and nurse to provide healthcare for sick community members. With support from the health project and small contributions (monthly premium) from community members, the CDC established a local health insurance scheme to cover the cost of treatment, including the salaries of medical staff. These initiatives demonstrate the power of community-led efforts in improving healthcare access and outcomes.

However, it is critical to entrust VDCs and VHCs with project related tasks only if they have proven their ability to perform them well, and if the PM and the project team find them to be reliable partners.[1]

The PM should keep in mind that VDCs and VHCs may sometimes have expectations for the project that it cannot meet. This is particularly true in remote communities where the nearest hospital may be far away. Community members and leaders may request that the project build a hospital in their village or provide patient transportation with project vehicles. However, fulfilling these demands may not align with the project's goals and objectives.

In these situations, communicating clearly with the committees and explaining what the project can do and what it cannot do is fruitful. For instance, the health project may not transport patients, but may be able to give them travel vouchers for traveling to a distant hospital for treatment. By coming up with creative solutions like this, the PM can show willingness to help while also clarifying to the VDCs and VHCs the project's mandate.

Religious leaders

Building strong relationships with leaders of the local church, mosques or temples can benefit the health project in several ways. Through partnering with religious leaders the PM can effectively promote health messages and provide healthcare-related information to their followers in support of the global health project. When the PM and their team treat them with respect and give them health information these religious leaders can widely spread these messages among their followers. During the 2013 to 2016 EVD epidemic in West Africa, many MOH agencies and NGOs partnered with local religious leaders to quickly spread key preventive messages in their communities. These leaders included in their regular sermons and preaching at churches and mosques the dos and don'ts for preventing the spread of the disease in their communities. It was an effective strategy.

> In the conservative northern Nigerian states of Sokoto, Niger, and Zamfara, Muslim religious leaders have been advocating for birth spacing and its benefits to their congregations. A local NGO educated these leaders on the significance of birth spacing and partnered with them to deliver messages on Family Planning topics during Friday sermons at mosques and counseling sessions.
>
> Conducting the End-of-Project evaluation, I found that the religious leaders had effectively educated their followers on this sensitive health topic in villages and towns where they had large followings. They utilized Friday prayer gatherings at mosques to openly teach the community members about the importance of spacing childbirth, yielding spectacular results.[2] Given the very conservative context it was not easy to achieve these results. But the health project was successful in improving Family Planning outcomes in communities by working with religious leaders.

Health projects can utilize places of worship for organizing important events, such as vaccination campaigns for children, distribution of food and health items, and venues where community health education can take place. These religious buildings and adjacent compounds can also serve as emergency shelters. Thus, developing and maintaining positive relationships with the religious leaders in the project community is crucial.

The MOH

There are four main models of interactions between the government organizations (MOH) and NGOs. Table 7.1 gives a summary of these models and their key features.

In certain LMICs, the MOH may lack the resources and funding necessary to plan and execute global health initiatives. To address this issue, NGO projects that receive funding from external donor agencies collaborate with the MOH to provide healthcare to the communities. Any of the four models listed in this table can be effective in achieving this goal.

For the success of the NGO health project the PM establishes a productive partnership with the MOH. They cultivate close working relationships with MOH representatives, including those at the sub-district, district, provincial, and national levels. Since MOH officials often have a high turnover rate due to frequent transfers, one needs to nurture personal and working relationships with them continually. Strong relationship is necessary not only with decision makers but also with junior staff members who may be responsible for releasing supplies to the project, such as safe delivery kits or Vitamin A.

Table 7.1 MOH–NGO interactions

Type	Partnering relationship	Key feature of partnership
Model 1	MOH and NGO implement a joint health project.	The two partners undertake separate complementary activities. E.g., MOH provides clinical services. NGO trains CHWs and volunteers for community mobilization.
Model 2	NGO sets up a project on its own, independent of the MOH.	NGO conducts its own project activities unhindered by government bureaucracy and responds to community needs. It must still liaise with the MOH and align with its goals.
Model 3	MOH contracts out healthcare services to NGO for local or district-wide implementation.	NGO manages health services in facilities and/or communities under MOH contract.
Model 4	MOH, NGO, private sector players, and businesses jointly implement large global health projects.	Some donors fund such coalition projects through a coordination mechanism. The coalition decides who will lead such a mechanism and negotiates the roles of each partner. Similar models with 'pooled funds' and multiple partners have been successful in many LMICs.

Many NGOs utilize MOH health facilities at various geographical levels for the project communities to access health services there. Models 1, 3, and 4 in Table 7.1 above allow NGOs to support tertiary and teaching hospitals, district hospitals and health centers, and sub-district health centers or health posts, as well as outreach programs. These three models not only enhance clinical healthcare services but also allow NGOs to conduct community mobilization and social and behavior change initiatives to improve community members' knowledge and practices. Additionally, NGOs can strengthen the MOH's supply chain management system for medicines and supplies. This is done through donation of these items to the MOH facilities and training the staff at these locations on the ordering, stocking, dispensing and waste disposal of medical supplies.

NGOs do not typically set up a parallel healthcare project of their own but instead assist the MOH in fulfilling its responsibilities, particularly in areas where there are shortcomings. Model 2 is the rare exception, where an NGO manages its own project with little involvement from MOH staff. However, it is uncommon nowadays to come across a model that functions completely independently of the MOH.

Sub-district or local level

This is where the health project team members would likely have most of their interactions with the MOH counterparts, especially when the project is focused on community health. The health project could be involved with training and supporting MOH midwives, nurses, and assistants stationed at health posts. The PM could assist these peripheral facilities with medicines and supplies and provide the workers there with health education materials for counseling or teaching community members on health topics. The team could also support MOH staff with record-keeping and reporting. If the project successfully develops and applies a new strategy in the project area, the PM can influence their MOH counterparts to accept this innovative strategy into their government health programming. However, the formal integration of an NGO strategy into the government system requires lobbying and approval at the district, provincial, or even national levels, which takes time and persistence.

District level

Mid-level MOH managers, technical staff, trainers, and logisticians are often based in district towns. These individuals are crucial decision-makers at the peripheral levels where your health project may be operating.

It is essential to establish a strong relationship with them and ensure they are familiar with the project.

There are various ways to interact with district-level MOH staff, including attending routine district meetings organized by the District Health Department. The PM may also request special meetings to present project objectives and progress, jointly solve problems, or obtain medical supplies for the project's health facilities or those government facilities supported by the health project.

There are trainers from MOH who work in specific districts and can train project staff or government facility staff on technical or administrative matters. For example, a district based MOH trainer can provide training on the latest preventive measures mandated by the government to reduce the spread of a disease in the community, or on how to record patient information in the health facilities and report it up the MOH chain of command. By facilitating such trainings, the project can empower government staff at the district and sub-district levels to carry out their tasks.

Supporting MOH district hospitals with medicine, supplies, and equipment can establish a positive relationship between facility staff and the project team. This relationship makes it easier for the team to refer patients from the project area to the district hospital for treatment. Additionally, the project team members may require treatment at these facilities, and positive impressions and bonds with the MOH staff there can lead to greater empathy towards the project teammates and patients from the project area.

In protracted emergency situations, the MOH may struggle to hire or retain skilled staff to run tertiary-level hospitals. In these cases, NGOs with skilled healthcare providers may be able to fill this gap and provide specialized healthcare at these facilities.

Once I came across a teaching hospital in a district of the Central African Republic that was affected by violent conflicts between ethnic groups for a prolonged period. Two international NGOs were jointly managing the surgical, maternity, pediatrics, and outpatient departments of the hospital with their own medical staff, because the MOH was unable to recruit medical professionals like surgeons, obstetricians, gynecologists, and pediatricians with the low government pay scale in that unstable region.

Provincial/regional and national level

Interactions with higher level MOH officials take place in large cities and national capitals. These interactions are usually meant to discuss policies, share information about the global health project, advocate for strategies that impact the project and the communities it serves, attend technical and management training, and resolve high-level issues. Securing approval for innovative approaches is also possible at these levels, which can then be integrated into MOH programming.

One effective way to garner support for the health project is to invite the high-level MOH officials to visit the project area and observe the activities and results in the communities.

The global health project I managed in Nagorno Karabakh focused on rehabilitating rural health centers that required significant repairs due to the damage caused by a recent war. Our project was responsible for reconstructing the buildings of several health centers. Once we completed the reconstruction of a set of village health centers, I invited the Minister for Health to join me and my team for the inauguration ceremony of these centers. We traveled to remote villages for a 'ribbon-cutting' ceremony at each newly reconstructed health center. News reporters and photojournalists accompanied us and covered the events widely. The Honorable Minister officially opened the centers, gave speeches, signed guest books, and appreciated the project's work and the opportunity to inaugurate these health centers.

Politicians in high positions often visit their constituencies to see for themselves and to showcase to others the positive development work that is being done in these places. These events are beneficial to both the MOH and the implementing agency and its projects, as they increase public awareness and visibility for both parties.

During emergencies like hurricanes, the MOH creates a national coordinating body for disaster response that involves various entities such as government agencies, international and national NGOs, donor organizations, and UN agencies. If the PM operates a health project in or near the disaster-stricken area, they may be asked to attend meetings and events related to the disaster response. If not invited, the PM needs to speak up and request that their organization and project be included. The PM comes prepared to these meetings, ready to give updates on the team's activities, provide local intelligence, and seek assistance for the project's response efforts. If the PM cannot attend, they should send a senior team member to such important meetings since the representation of the project and the implementing organization is of vital importance.

While some may view these activities as distractions from the project's primary goals, collaborating with others in the disaster response and relief activities not only contributes to humanitarian efforts in the project area but also demonstrates that the PM and their team are reliable partners during emergencies. This, in turn, can enhance the health project's reputation and lead to new partnerships with implementing and donor organizations.

In an emergency situation, the government often reaches out to large NGOs for assistance. They may urgently request the temporary use of NGO vehicles, storage spaces, or other assets. If the PM receives such a request from the MOH or other government ministries, they may need to temporarily release one or more of their project vehicles for disaster relief operations, as an example. Before deciding, however, one should review the organization's policies and practices and consult with senior staff and supervisors to determine the appropriate response. There must be good planning and preparations made ahead of time for responding to such unexpected requests so there are alternative strategies in place to continue with the health project work in case some of the project assets are tied up in an emergency for an extended period of time.

Other non-health government ministries

In addition to the MOH, there are other government ministries with which one would want to establish partnerships. For instance, your global health project may involve school health activities, nutrition-related interventions, or collaboration with religious leaders and places of worship. In such cases, the project may require approval from the ministries of education, agriculture, religious affairs, and others in some LMICs. Also, officials from these ministries may express interest in visiting the project sites to better understand how health benefits can be delivered to communities through non-health structures and systems. Therefore, it is beneficial to establish relationships with representatives from these non-health ministries at all levels.

Non-government voluntary agencies

In areas where the global health project is located, NGOs, FBOs, and CBOs can emerge as valuable partners. Unfortunately, some PMs view these organizations as competitors rather than potential collaborators, and remain uninterested in building any relationship with them, which is a missed opportunity. Experienced leaders understand the benefits of working together, even when these organizations operate in non-health sectors.

There are several ways the PM and their team can collaborate with these organizations. They might organize cross-visits to share best practices and learn from each other. Also, PMs sometimes develop a protocol for sharing medical supplies, transport, and equipment with other NGOs. If these organizations have health facilities in or near the project areas, the team encourages project community members and staff to seek treatment there. Additionally, in case of a disaster, the PM pools resources with these organizations to set up a joint response in the project communities.

To foster a sense of community, collaborative PMs consider organizing social events that bring together team members from different agencies. This helps break down barriers and increase camaraderie among everyone involved.

One time while traveling in Uganda, I had the opportunity to attend a social gathering organized by the PM of our organization's health project. These gatherings occurred once a month on weekends and brought together project team members, colleagues from other national and international NGOs, representatives from the donor organization, and staff from the MOH office. The atmosphere was filled with music, laughter, and delicious food, creating a special bonding experience for everyone.

I discovered that many attendees looked forward to these monthly gatherings as they provided a break from the routine stress of project work. The PM in Uganda was praised for creating this opportunity for individuals to de-stress and socialize outside of work, breaking down barriers and promoting better teamwork. The support the PM received from all parties involved was tremendous, resulting in positive outcomes and good rapport for the project.

When collaborating with other NGOs, the experienced PM ensures that their principles and ethics are aligned with those of the project implementing organization. One carefully examines their policies and practices regarding the use of tobacco, weapons, and products that harm the environment. For instance, the PM might find that an NGO promotes the use of breast milk substitutes for infants, or that its staff at the health center do not treat women with respect, or there are doubts about its motivation or financial practices. Their political affiliation can be problematic as well. Thus, it is prudent to exercise caution and due diligence before entering into a formal partnership with such organizations.

Additionally, the PM establishes a clear understanding of each organization's roles and geographical areas of project operation to avoid overlapping or encroaching on each other's work. They avoid duplicating efforts of building two adjacent health centers on the same project site and competing for patients, for example. Instead, organizations can collaborate and pool their resources to operate a larger facility and share patient care responsibilities. Alternatively, they could explore the need to build and operate such facilities in different locations to meet a greater need and provide wider coverage.

UN organizations

Having close relationships with UN agencies in the country can be advantageous for a health project. Some UN agencies fund certain project activities. For example, UNHCR often funds projects that work with refugees and WFP offers financial and material aid in crisis situations. Additionally, WHO and UNICEF offices in the project country or their regional offices offer a wealth of technical information and support.

During humanitarian emergencies, UN organizations and other agencies, such as government bodies, NGOs, the Red Cross/Red Crescent Movement, donor agencies, and other humanitarian organizations establish "clusters" that work in specific technical sectors like health, water and sanitation, and protection. If a natural or human caused disaster occurs in the project area and clusters are activated in response, the PM or their delegates attend the cluster meetings to contribute to the response efforts, particularly in the health cluster. Offering resources to other related clusters also helps the health project communities overcome disaster-related losses and promotes the project and its organization to other partners in the clusters.

Humanitarian crisis can arise from armed conflicts among population groups. Often the UN Peacekeeping forces become activated to keep civilians safe in a crisis setting. If the health project operates in such a volatile setting, it is a good idea to build close contacts with the officials in the locally deployed UN Peacekeeping force so they can offer the project staff adequate protection and advice against atrocities if there is a need.

Funding agencies

Donor agencies are interested in partnering with NGOs to fund the implementation of their projects. However, they must ensure that their implementing partners operate within the agreed rules and regulations. Therefore, they require routine project reports, including financial reports from the health project. Donors must raise funds from their own financial supporters and provide them with project updates and facts. Thus, they depend on the PM's timely submission of project progress and financial reports.

Reporting to donors should not be seen as a burden. Providing complete and timely reports and discussing any challenges faced by the project will build donor confidence in the project and its implementing organization. Responding promptly to any queries from donors and keeping them informed of any significant changes in project strategies and expenses will strengthen the trust and commitment they have in the project.

When there is a need the PM does not hesitate to meet with donors and their team members at their local office to discuss project progress or important issues. Donors may organize training programs on new rules and regulations or reporting procedures that recipient organizations must follow. There may be new funding available which the donor organizations want to discuss with their existing project partners. The PM takes advantage of these opportunities and attends these events personally or delegates a senior team member to participate. Keeping close cooperation with donors helps with managing the health project effectively.

Donor agency staff may want to visit the project sites to monitor activities. The experienced PM always receives them cordially at the project offices and sites and share both the project's achievements and challenges with them. They can give valuable advice and help make accommodations if necessary.

If the implementing organization is seeking new funding for future project phases the likelihood of securing potential grants is high when the PM maintains a strong collaborative relationship with the current donor. It is also worth considering connecting with other funding agencies in the country where the project operates, as they may become possible future donors.

Sometimes a donor agency may try to dictate the way a project should function, which can be problematic. A wise PM resists the pressure or temptation to become "donor-driven" and instead cultivates a frank and collegial relationship with donors from the beginning. Such a relationship can be useful in preventing micro-management by the donors, educating the donors, and negotiating with them. It is also wise to diversify the donor base and explore funding from multiple sources.

Private sector practitioners, and facilities

Engaging with this particular set of external stakeholders can be challenging, especially when it comes to protecting project communities from harmful practices of traditional healers while also turning such private practitioners into allies. To achieve this, the PM and their team establish personal relationships with them, explaining the project's goals, offering them with training on modern health practices, avoiding public criticism, and involving them in the global health project. Additionally, the PM considers including them in the team's training sessions, providing them with relevant educational materials, and helping them access online webinars and conferences on global health topics. In most cases they feel proud to be exposed to modern healthcare. By embracing these strategies, the PM fosters positive collaborations that benefit the project communities.

Financial institutions

Many banks and credit unions offer local community members soft loans with low interest rates. This helps the loan recipients for instance to run small businesses to supplement their income. If the project has an intervention to help the community members to borrow money to start a small business, one could link them up to a lending institution operating in the project area. Community members can be financially stronger and physically healthier utilizing the profit they make from their businesses. They can use this fund to do home repairs, buy food for their children, or pay for transportation to the health center for medical care, to give a few examples.

In monitoring a large project spanning multiple regions in Ethiopia, I visited the project team that had formed small groups of HIV-positive individuals in rural communities. With the project's help these groups were able to secure soft loans for small businesses through arrangements made with local banks. The project provided support to recipients of these loans to start their own cooperative businesses. For example, one group established a small chicken farm that produced enough chicken and eggs to improve their own nutrition and sell them in the local market for a profit. This resulted in an improvement in their finances as well. Another group raised goats and sheep for the same purpose fetching similar results.

Other groups used their loan funds to start village stores in their community and earned enough profits to purchase nutritious food

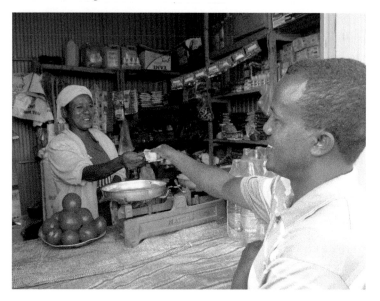

Image 7.2 Local store run by a person with HIV+ status in Ethiopia

and other items for their families. Due to the strong stigma in the community against individuals with HIV and the lack of privacy of their status, it was challenging for them to find employment. This soft loan scheme was significant in improving the income, nutrition, and self-esteem of the HIV-positive community members that partnered with the project. Image 7.2 captures a success story.

Key takeaways

- There are important interactions a PM can have with external stakeholders. These entities have an interest in the global health project and can affect the project or be affected by the project outcomes.
- For engaging community members and leaders, the PM might organize large open-air community meetings or smaller meetings respectively.
- VDCs and VHCs (also CDCs and CHCs) can provide great support and valuable advice to a global health project. Particularly, VHCs and CHCs can be instrumental in assisting the project.
- If such a grass root committee does not exist or is inactive explore with the community leaders and members ways to reactivate or establish these committees, particularly the VHC or CHC.

- Religious leaders can be effective in spreading health messages. They can offer their places of worship for project work.
- The MOH often has gaps which a donor funded NGO can bridge in collaboration with the MOH staff at all levels. There are at least four models of interactions between NGOs and the MOH.
- NGOs can assist the MOH in the areas of healthcare services as well as community mobilization. Training and mentoring MOH staff, as well as utilizing MOH trainers to train the health project staff can be a productive collaboration.
- NGOs normally do not set up parallel healthcare systems or projects but assist the MOH to perform its mandate.
- In policy discussions and for lobbying purposes an NGO might interact with the MOH at the national or provincial level. Humanitarian crisis often brings together the MOH and NGOs along with other agencies. The PM should actively participate in 'cluster' activities during such an emergency.
- Collaboration with other NGOs, FBOs, and CBOs can bring rewarding experiences. Making cross-visits, sharing costly equipment and transportation, and aiding with medical supplies are a few examples of effective interactions between these agencies and the project.
- Enjoying social time with the staff of external organizations gives the project team an opportunity to build close relationships with them outside of working hours.
- The experienced PM is vigilant about counterproductive and unethical principles and practices that some external organizations might adopt. They enter into formal relationships only after doing due diligence.
- It is beneficial to maintain close contacts with UN organizations. Often funds, material aid, technical information, and protection are offered by UN organizations to NGO projects.
- Donor organizations require timely and complete technical and financial reports from projects they fund. Frank discussion of issues related to project performance, arrangement for project site visits, and attending meetings with donors are quite productive.
- Undue pressure from or micromanaging the health project by a donor agency should be resisted and resolved with frank and collegial discussions.
- Establishing personal relationships with traditional health practitioners, pharmacists, and village midwives; explaining to them the health project's intended benefits for the communities; and engaging them in project activities can help build good rapport with these private sector practitioners and secure their cooperation.

Discussion questions

1. What are the benefits of a collaborative relationship between a health project and the VHC?
2. Which of the four models of MOH-NGO interactions is your preference, and why?
3. Why is it important to maintain close collaboration with donor agencies?
4. What are the benefits and risks of partnering with other NGOs similar to yours?
5. How can UN agencies working in your project country or location assist your health project?
6. True or false questions: For each numbered statement in Table 7.2 write 'T' or 'F' to indicate 'True' or 'False' respectively.

Table 7.2 True or false questions

No.	Statement	T / F
1.	External stakeholders can include local communities, government (MOH) offices, and donor agencies supporting the health project.	
2.	Communities always have active committees that work to benefit the people.	
3.	Religious leaders are preoccupied with spiritual ministries, and they are never interested in health matters. Thus, they are not ideal partners for a health project.	
4.	For a health project to be successful it is important to maintain close relationships with the local MOH.	
5.	Traditional healers, village doctors and pharmacists, and traditional birth attendants often do not correctly practice medicine. Yet they are quite popular in their communities.	
6.	The PM should never inform the donor agencies about any issues with project implementation or budget because funding for the project may stop.	

See correct answers on page 194.

Case study exercise

Imagine you are the PM of an immunization project operated by an NGO in Bangladesh. Your team has developed an innovative strategy to enhance the MOH immunization efforts. The approach involves (i) routine monitoring of CHWs by MOH supervisors, (ii) compilation of supervision findings, and (iii) monthly training of CHWs based on the supervision results. The innovative strategy has proven effective, and MOH staff and managers at the sub-district and district levels are willing to integrate it into their immunization program. However, they require formal approval from the MOH at regional and national levels to implement this strategy. What steps will you and your team take to help get the necessary approval and integrate this effective approach into the MOH program protocol?

See Author's suggestion on page 198–199.

Notes

1 Ted Lankester, "Setting up Environmental Health Improvements," in *Setting Up Community Health Programmes* (Berkeley, Hesperian, 2009).
2 The Mitchell Group, Inc., "The Leadership Development for Family Planning / Reproductive Health For Political Office Holders, Traditional and Religious Leaders Project," *USAID|Nigeria's Monitoring and Evaluation Project II (MEMS II)*, February 12, 2014, accessed May 15, 2023, https://pdf.usaid.gov/pdf_docs/PA00JP52.pdf

References

Lankester, Ted. 2009. "Setting up Environmental Health improvements," in *Setting Up Community Health Programmes*. Berkeley: Hesperian.
The Mitchell Group, Inc. 2014. "The Leadership Development for Family Planning/Reproductive Health For Political Office Holders, Traditional and Religious Leaders Project." *USAID|Nigeria's Monitoring and Evaluation Project II (MEMS II)*. February 12, 2014. Accessed May 15, 2023. https://pdf.usaid.gov/pdf_docs/PA00JP52.pdf

8   Managing project budgets

Implementing a health project, whether big or small, requires funding to cover various tasks and subtasks, as well as purchases of necessary items such as medical supplies, building materials for health centers, mosquito nets, hygienic latrine components, vehicles, and more, all depending on the project's objectives. Additionally, there are expenses related to staff salaries, office rent, travel, utilities, and many other costs necessary to run a health project. Generally, in LMICs, donor agencies provide funding for project expenses, and they require a high degree of fiscal transparency and integrity in the use of their funds. A successful project is typically the one that has a practical budget developed, a functional budget tracking system, and which the PM completes within the allocated funds.

In this chapter, we will discuss the process of creating and overseeing project budgets, as well as the most effective techniques for fiscal management. The PM is responsible for two basic tasks when it comes to managing project funds: developing the budget and tracking expenses. However, it is typical for others within the implementing organization and/or the health project itself (team members with finance background) to assist the PM with these responsibilities. Whether one manages a government health project under the MOH or an NGO-operated project they will have an operating budget, and they will ensure that project funds are used in accordance with that budget.

Developing project budgets

A project budget is a comprehensive estimation of the total cost involved in completing a project with high quality within a specified time frame. It outlines the amount of money the project will spend, what it will be spent on, and when it will be spent. By preparing a budget plan and monitoring the spending throughout the project life, the PM can minimize the risk of running out of funds or having surplus funds when the project ends.

Here are the essential steps for developing a project budget.

DOI: 10.4324/9781003405245-9

Getting support from the finance department

Almost all implementing agencies (MOH or NGOs) will have a finance department that oversees all financial matters including budget development and expenditure tracking of projects. It is quite likely that the project implementing agency will provide support and advice to the PM for developing and tracking budgets for the health project through its finance department. The department may have its experienced staff at the organizational headquarters, its regional offices, and in the country office where the PM is usually based. In a large project, the PM may have one or more finance persons on their health project team that are placed there from the finance department.

For assisting the PM with developing and tracking the project budget, the finance department colleagues will require specific cost information on the project to perform these functions accurately. In both government and NGO health projects, the information the team provides ultimately reaches the finance department at headquarters, where colleagues with a finance background will review, finalize, and approve the project budget. The accuracy of the project budget depends on the correct cost information the PM and their team provide to the finance department. For example, the project budget may need to include the cost of printing health education materials locally, or the expense of fuel purchases for project vehicles. The project team along with the PM is most knowledgeable for providing the correct information on these expenses because they are most familiar with these expenditures. Providing accurate cost information to the finance department will help them draw up a budget for the project that is practical and useful.

Using a budget template

There is usually a budget template that the finance department shares with the PM in the field that helps in collecting and transmitting the estimated cost of budget items. It is normally a blank template with guidance for the PM to include a detailed estimate of all costs that the project is likely to incur during its life. Usually, large organizations will want all their PMs to use a standardized template throughout the organization for ease of financial analysis and reporting across all projects. In the absence of such a standard template, PMs create a budget template using a software package or build their own custom template suitable for their projects. A budget template generally includes these broad categories of project expenditures:

- Employee salaries and wages – for all expatriate and local staff working on the project.
- Employee benefits – fringe benefits for staff as appropriate and according to organization policies.

- Consultant fees – for internal and external experts supporting the project.
- Travel expenses – for domestic and international airfare, accommodation, per diem, visas, airport taxes, and local transport.
- Equipment costs – project vehicles, computers, printers, cameras.
- Supplies – office supplies, postage, and mailing.
- Contractual fees – for subcontractors and vendors that work for or support the project.
- Project interventions – specific expenses for conducting planned interventions.
- Other direct costs – vehicle fuel, storage rent, electricity, communications (internet, phones, faxes), generator, and security services.
- Indirect cost – usually a certain percentage of the direct costs agreed upon with the funding agency. Sometimes referred to as Negotiated Indirect Cost Rate Agreement, these indirect costs are related to overhead expenditures such as utilities, rent, and insurance, etc., that are in addition to direct costs.[1]

The list above is not exhaustive, but it provides an idea of expenses that the project team and PM should submit to the finance department on the detailed budget template. These expenses are linked to project objectives and activities along with a timeline. Therefore, the budget plan displays how expenses are to be made for attaining each project objective and breaks the budget into time periods, such as monthly, quarterly, or half-yearly. It is beneficial to determine how much funding is allocated for specific objectives and how much is used over a certain period. The PM and finance department require this level of detail for tracking financial performance throughout the project.

Reviewing the project activity plan

Budgets are tied to project goals, objectives, tasks, sub-tasks, and deadlines. For developing a practical budget, one needs to refer to each of these. To give an example, the number of latrines or water pumps that will be installed in the project area, the number of weeks or months the installation will take, and the cost of material and labor will all determine the line item cost estimate in the project's budget for latrine and water pump installation. Ideally the DAP should have project activities planned out in details, as we discussed in chapter 3. So, reviewing these plans for project activities in the DAP helps in estimating the expenses for these activities.

Determining the resources needed

When compiling a list of project deliverables – including tasks like installing latrines and water pumps – one should identify all the necessary resources. These resources come with associated costs, such as the wages of project team members, materials, equipment, travel, and training. The PM creates a comprehensive list to ensure no costs are overlooked. Again, each resource should be linked to a strong rationale for including it in the budget. If a cost, such as purchasing additional vehicles, does not contribute to the project's objectives, it is unlikely to be approved by the finance department and senior management.

Calculating the cost of each resource

The unit cost of each resource that is listed in the previous step must be well understood and used for calculating the total cost. Note that all staff will not cost the same, with more experienced team members having a higher salary than junior staff or those hired more recently. Materials, contractors, and vendors also have varying rates. The PM recognizes the costs at different project sites may vary.

Estimating the total cost for all project activities

Once the PM has considered the necessary resources and their costs, they create a budget estimate for each resource. If the project is new, or if the PM is new to the project, the information included in the budget template may be an estimate. However, if the PM has previously worked on a similar project, they use their experience to determine the costs of resources in the budget line items. Alternatively, the PM and their team make an educated guess about the budget line item costs. In either case, the information one provides to the finance department will help them develop what is often called a 'ballpark estimate.'

Including contingency fund

When estimating the total expenses for a project, it is difficult to predict any potential cost increases over the life of the project with complete certainty. This is especially true for large, complex projects that span multiple years and involve multiple interventions. There are many factors that can contribute to increased costs, such as inflation, fluctuations in currency exchange rates, and changes in political and economic conditions. For this reason, it is wise to allocate approximately ten percent of the total budget as a reserve fund for emergencies. Some organizations may not prioritize the inclusion of such a fund, as they aim to make their budget as accurate as possible. The PM collaborates with colleagues in the finance department to determine how to budget for unexpected expenses.

Drafting the project budget

To create a project budget, the PM uses the budget template from the finance department or a software program to compile the estimated cost of the project. If there is room in the template, one should include the rationale for the costs, especially for the big ticket line items as well as the assumptions, risks, and timelines for major project activities.

Once the draft budget is ready, the PM shares it with senior team members, particularly those who oversee the project's finances. Their feedback can help detect any omission or error. The draft budget is then refined and improved before submitting it for approval. The PM ensures all necessary expenses are included in the draft budget for successful project implementation.

Submitting budget for approval

After completing the draft budget, the PM submits it to the finance department in the prescribed format, or any other acceptable format if the department does not furnish a template. The PM includes notes and other necessary paperwork in the submission. The finance department reviews the proposed budget along with supporting documents, requests clarifications if necessary, negotiates certain costs with the PM, and obtains the final budget approval.

Modifying project budget as needed

Budgeting is an important part of project management, and the budget is not a fixed financial plan. Instead, it needs to be continually assessed and modified throughout the project's lifecycle with input from finance department colleagues and the project team. As the project progresses, the budget is adjusted to reflect more refined and accurate estimates. Finance department colleagues often refer to this as the rough order of magnitude (ROM) estimate, which they periodically share with the PM.

To summarize the discussion above, for managing a project budget effectively, the PM and their team gather unit prices for all expenses and use a budget template to calculate costs for each item. This draft budget is then submitted to the finance department for approval and release of funds. Throughout the project, the PM monitors expenses with the support of their team and finance department colleagues, making necessary modifications and adjustments to the budget and project activities. If the

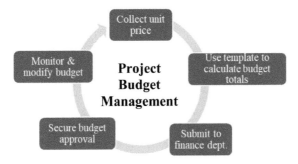

Figure 8.1 Project budget management cycle

project expands or is implemented over additional years, new budgets are developed.

Thus, project budget management involves a cyclical process of assessing costs, modifying budgets, and monitoring project expenses. The sequential steps of this process are detailed in Figure 8.1.

Monitoring project budget

As mentioned earlier the PM is responsible not only for creating project budgets, but also for monitoring them. This involves keeping a close watch on project expenses to ensure they remain within budget.

Projects rarely go exactly as planned. The PM should regularly review project expenses to identify any deviations from the budget. Such a deviation is known as 'budget vs. actual' (BvA) variance, and it can be detected by tracking and analyzing project expenses.

By routinely tracking expenses and comparing them to the budget, one can quickly identify any instances where costs tend to exceed budgeted amounts or remain lower than the budget. If this occurs, the PM and their team members should investigate the causes and make necessary adjustments before the costs significantly deviate from the budget amount. If there is deviation the PM includes the BvA variance in the financial reports that they send to the finance department and other stakeholders.

Regular expense tracking can also alert the PM about the need for additional funds to cover a particular line item in the budget. By identifying this need early in the project, the PM avoids delays or disruptions in project activities while trying to secure additional funds. Therefore, monitoring project expenses and comparing them to budget amounts for each line item is essential in detecting BvA variance.

> While managing the global health project in Nagorno Karabakh, I held monthly meetings with the finance manager of my organization to review project expenditures. The project had a detailed budget that allocated funds for each task and sub-task.
>
> Over the course of several months, we both noticed that one specific line item was consistently exceeding its monthly budget. This was the cost of transporting medicines and supplies to the twenty plus far-flung health centers that the project supported. When we asked the driver of the truck about the high expense, he explained that his truck frequently blew out its tires on the rough mountain terrain, and his cost of replacing these tires was very high. While there were receipts to support his claims, I had a strong suspicion that his explanation was not really genuine.
>
> To address the issue, I considered finding a less expensive vendor to replace the current driver. However, when the current driver learned about my intentions, he promised to reduce this cost and requested that his contract not be terminated. I honored his request, and to my pleasant surprise, the cost of trucking the medical supplies immediately returned to normal! While there were still some genuine tire purchases throughout the remainder of the project, the expense was within a reasonable range. As a result, the transportation line item did not exceed its total annual budget, and the project was able to complete its course without any over-expenditure. I was grateful that we were able to detect and address the issue early in the project's life.
>
> If it weren't for the diligent expense review process and the thorough record-keeping skills of the finance manager, the project would have been in dire straits due to the excessively high monthly expenditure of just one budget line item.

There are many causes for BvA variance.

- Underestimating budget line item costs.
- Using unrealistic cost estimates.
- Misjudging the intricacies of project activities.
- Miscalculating project schedule.
- Neglecting to consider contingencies and emergencies.
- Lacking experience in budgeting.

The need to address these causes right from the beginning of the project cannot be overemphasized.

Managing budget overrun

A budget overrun occurs when the actual cost of a project exceeds the initially planned budget. It can also happen when a project is operated beyond the established deadline, which affects the project's cost performance.[2] Keeping track of expenses can help the PM identify unforeseen factors that may later cause financial problems for the project. By doing so, one can address these issues early on preventing them from becoming difficult to resolve later.

When the experienced PM faces a budget overrun, they take the following actions:

- Requests additional funds from senior management and the finance department, providing valid reasons along with plans to control project expenses.
- Utilizes unused or underused funds from one line item to cover the cost of the more expensive line item that is causing the budget overrun.
- Improves project efficiency.
- Defers certain project activities to future projects, reduces project activities, or removes them altogether from the project plan if necessary.
- Lowers the volume of project services and deliverables.
- Uses lower-cost resources instead of more expensive ones. For example, considers online training for project staff instead of organizing more costly in-person training, or uses less expensive junior staff to perform tasks that higher-paid project staff would typically handle.
- Uses contingency funds in the project budget to cover deficits, but only if all other attempts to control expenses have failed.

A word of caution and advice on managing project budgets

In global health project management one of the most challenging and critical tasks is managing the project budget. Even if a PM completes the project on time and achieves exceptional results with significant improvement of community health, overspending the allocated budget funds is interpreted as a failure.

To avoid such disasters, it is essential for the PM to continually improve their budgeting skills throughout their career in project management. PMs need not hesitate to ask for guidance from experienced colleagues, especially those in the finance department. Looking for mentors both within and outside their organization who can support the PM is a smart thing to do. Expanding one's knowledge of managing project budgets by studying publications can be fruitful. The PM can join online or in-person groups that discuss the latest thinking on project management and budgeting, so they can learn, ask questions, and contribute to the discussions.

With sincere efforts PMs can reap rich rewards. Delivering excellent results while successfully controlling project costs can lead to great career potential.

Key takeaways

- The budget is an effective management tool to assess if the project is on track for meeting its goals within the planned funding.
- A project budget is the total estimated cost that details how much will be spent, for what, and by when so the PM can complete the project on time and with high quality.
- The PM develops and controls the project budget with support from colleagues in the finance department. A successful project is one that is completed within the allocated funds.
- The finance department needs from the PM certain information so it can help develop and track the project budget. The PM and their team members are the most informed on field level expenses, and so they should provide the cost information to their finance colleagues.
- Budget is created using a template that includes all categories of project expenditures.
- It is wise to build into the budget a contingency (reserve) fund of around ten percent of the total budget for emergencies.
- The project budget is not a static financial plan. It is continuously reviewed and revised based on ongoing expenditures.
- The PM periodically reviews the budget to detect BvA variance, making it possible for early detection of any deviation and quick remedy of any issues.
- Budget overruns occur when expenses exceed the budget.
- One of several ways to address budget overruns is to use contingency funds to cover deficits. But this fund should be utilized only if absolutely necessary, and when all other measures have failed.
- Far-sighted PMs continuously improve their budgeting skills as they build their project management career. This takes hard work, but their sincere efforts can yield rich rewards.

Discussion questions

1. What are the elements of the project budget management cycle?
2. Why is it crucial for a PM to regularly review project expenses?
3. What can be some reasons for a health project to overspend its budget?
4. Do you believe that developing and controlling the project budget is a critical management skill for a PM? Why or why not?

5. True or false questions: For each numbered statement in Table 8.1 write 'T' or 'F' to indicate 'True' or 'False' respectively.

Table 8.1 True or false questions

No.	Statement	T / F
1.	A project budget is the estimated total cost involved in completing a project.	
2.	The PM should seek support from the finance department in developing project budgets and tracking expenses.	
3.	In developing project budgets reviewing the DAP is necessary as budgets are linked to project activities.	
4.	A project budget is a final document and should not be modified during the project's life.	
5.	The PM monitors the BvA to detect under- or over-expenditures of budget line items.	
6.	One way to manage budget overruns is to increase the volume of project activities and deliverables.	

See correct answers on page 194.

Case study exercise

Imagine you are the PM of a global health project in an LMIC. While reviewing the project's monthly expenses, you observe that some of the cost items have exceeded the allocated budget by a significant amount. Happily, you have identified this BvA variance early in the project's life. What actions can you take to rectify this budget overrun and get the project back on track within the budget?

See Author's suggestion on page 199.

Notes

1 Alicia Tuovila, "Overhead: What it Means in Business, Major Types, and Examples," *Investopedia,* Updated August 23, 2022, www.investopedia.com/terms/o/overhead.asp

2 Naveen Ilangovan, "Keeping your project on budget and avoiding project overruns," *Technical skills* (blog), *Australian Institute of Project Management,* January 23, 2020, https://aipm.com.au/blog/keeping-your-project-on-budget/

References

Ilangovan, Naveen. 2020. "Keeping your project on budget and avoiding project overruns." *Technical skills* (blog). *Australian Institute of Project Management.* January 23. https://aipm.com.au/blog/keeping-your-project-on-budget/

Tuovila, Alicia. 2022. "Overhead: What it Means in Business, Major Types, and Examples." *Investopedia.* August 23. Accessed May 31, 2023. www.investopedia.com/terms/o/overhead.asp

9 Monitoring health project activities

During a five-year MNCH project operated by an NGO in Central Asia, there were delays in many project activities over the initial year and a half of implementation. The newly appointed PM was pre-occupied with attending meetings and conferences, and engaging in various activities, but did not ensure the completion of project tasks and sub-tasks despite having a detailed plan in place. The PM failed to follow this plan, nor did he monitor the activities, thus hindering the project's progress. Staff recruitment was delayed, procurement of project vehicles did not occur promptly, and health education sessions for caregivers of children were stalled, resulting in the project budget remaining underspent for over a year. As the headquarters-based senior advisor and manager of this project I began to notice this delay when I started to monitor the project remotely.

The donor organization and senior management at the head-quarters were anxious to see the project perform according to plans. Through monitoring visits, some changes were made in the field, and the project's implementation began to improve.

This improvement was possible because headquarters staff began monitoring the project, albeit somewhat late in the project cycle. Typically, the PM stationed in-country should diligently monitor the project so that all its planned tasks and sub-tasks proceed according to plan.

Purpose of global health project monitoring

In the previous chapter we discussed among other things, the importance of routinely monitoring project expenses and comparing them to the project budget. Here, we will discuss the monitoring of project progress, which in principle is quite similar to monitoring project budget.

The process of monitoring project progress involves tracking its planned activities over time. For instance, a water and sanitation project aims to install a specific number of hand pumps within a set timeframe to provide safe drinking water for the community. As the project is carried

DOI: 10.4324/9781003405245-10

out, the PM must ensure that the installation of these pumps is following the detailed plan for this activity. Monitoring the project regularly not only tracks its progress, but also helps identify potential difficulties or delays with tasks or sub-tasks that could hinder project completion.

To use that same example above, if monitoring detects a delay in the installation of water pumps, then the team can find alternative ways to complete the task on time. Delays can be caused by various factors, such as suppliers failing to deliver the pumps on time or local workers from the project community threatening to stop working unless their demand for more pay is met. In each of these scenarios, the PM and the team must find suitable solutions quickly to keep the project on schedule. To address any issues with pumps delivery and workers' remuneration, it may be necessary to look for a new supplier and seek assistance from community leaders. Early detection of delays or problems with project activities allows the PM and the project team to take corrective measures sooner rather than later. Without proper monitoring delays or problems may go unnoticed and cause the project to fall behind schedule and not meet its goals. Therefore, it is important to routinely track project tasks to quickly identify and address any potential issues.

In addition to checking on activities and taking corrective actions, monitoring also has another critical use in global health projects. The PM submits regular reports to senior managers in the organization, who in turn submit donor reports to the funding agencies that support the project. These reports include an important section on project progress, which senior management and donors review to determine what has been accomplished, what tasks are falling behind, and what is being done to speed up progress. Thus, monitoring is necessary for gathering activity data to prepare project progress reports.

Developing and using indicators to track project progress

Indicators are tools that help measure progress. Just as a yardstick is used to measure the length of a table or the height of a wall, indicators are used to measure the success of a global health project. For instance, in a water and sanitation project, an indicator could be the number of hand pumps installed or the number of households that use these pumps. Similarly, in a maternal health project, the number of births that take place in a health facility is a powerful indicator. In a COVID-19 control project, a useful indicator to track would be the number of people who have received recommended vaccines.

Global health projects use various indicators to measure their progress, including quantitative indicators that monitor *numbers* related to tasks and sub-tasks. These numbers are compared to targets set by the project for achieving specific outputs over a set period. This period may be a month, quarter, six-month period, a year, and the entire project life. Thus, the targets are reference points or mile markers set for these time periods.

Indicators that measure numbers are called *quantitative* indicators. There are also *qualitative* methods that measure project progress differently. Since qualitative assessment takes a relatively longer time and more resources, it is often reserved for project evaluations that take place only at specific points in the project's life. Evaluation methodologies including qualitative assessments are covered in the following chapter.

To use the water and sanitation examples above it is worth noting that indicators can vary in type, measuring either project *outputs* or *outcomes*. See Chapter 1 for discussion on project input, output, and outcome.

Output indicators

When a project installs water pumps in the community, the *number* of pumps it installs is considered its output. For instance, if a project successfully installed 100 pumps in a year in an urban slum community, its output for that year would be 100 pumps. The number of installed pumps is the *direct* and *immediate* result of the project's activity, which is the installation of water pumps at the project sites.

To measure the progress of the project, the 'number of hand pumps installed' should be used as an output indicator. This activity can be monitored monthly or quarterly by observing and documenting the number of pumps installed. When the monitors use this output indicator, the PM can find in their monitoring reports a clear picture of the progress made in hand pump installation.

To keep track of progress, the team should set targets for each output at the beginning of the project and compare these outputs against the set targets every month or quarter. This comparison will help to determine whether the project is on schedule and whether any specific site is underperforming. Using output indicators routinely for monitoring project tasks enables the PM to take corrective actions quickly if needed, without having to wait until a later stage of the project, when it may be difficult or impossible to fix any underlying issues.

Outcome indicators

Different from output indicators are the *outcome* indicators in that these do not measure the numbers of direct results that the project is achieving, items it is distributing, or events it is organizing. The monitors use outcome indicators to still count numbers, but these numbers reflect the *change* that the project has brought about in the communities. These changes are *indirect* and *longer term* in nature.

Prior to the start of the health project, let us imagine the community members lacked or had only limited access to safe drinking water. However, since the installation of the hand pumps, they are now able to use safe water from these pumps for drinking and cooking. This is *change* – positive change – in the community. It is an *indirect* result of the project activity (installing the hand pumps). To measure the outcomes of the project, one uses outcome indicators, such as the 'number of households or individuals consuming water from the installed hand pumps.'

Other examples of outcome indicators include the number of individuals that are sleeping under mosquito bed nets (as opposed to the number of bed nets distributed, which is an output indicator). Also, the number of births that took place in a health center. This would be a major change in the community where most births probably used to take place at homes before the health project started, increasing the risk of maternal and neonatal mortality and morbidity.

However, for routine monitoring that takes place each month or quarter most projects do not assess the outcomes of the project. It would need significant time and funds to undertake outcome monitoring frequently. Thus, the measuring of outcomes is usually performed through project evaluations at set intervals in the project's life, normally, at the beginning, mid-point and at the end of a project. The following chapter gives details on project evaluations.

Input indicators

In addition to output and outcome indicators, there are input indicators that measure the utilization of resources for project activities. These resources primarily include funding, but can also include staff, vehicles, computers, and furniture. It is critical to closely track project resources that are being spent to ensure they align with project activity plans and budget.

Understanding the reasons for input changes and discussing them in the project report to senior management along with the steps taken to manage these changes is important.

The process of monitoring global health projects

Ideally, the health project monitoring begins at the planning stage with the setting up of indicators for project outputs, outcomes, and inputs. This is done when the project team develops the project's DAP, which has been covered in Chapter 3.

Documenting indicators and means of verification

The DAP usually documents the indicators and targets for each activity. Additionally, it should identify the *sources* from which information about the indicators can be obtained, also known as the 'means of verification.' If this is not done at that DAP stage, the project team, should select these before beginning the monitoring of the project. The PM and their team must create a usable format with these elements for monitoring the project outputs.

Selecting project monitors

In many health projects, those senior team members who supervise and support the junior staff are responsible for routine monitoring. They receive training on how to use indicators, targets, and means of verification to assess the project outputs that result from the tasks and sub-tasks.

In an LMIC setting where the MOH operates multiple projects across the country, a dedicated team of staff with monitoring and evaluation skills may be housed within the MOH. In the case of an implementing NGO this team may be located in its country office, or in its regional or international headquarters. This team is often referred to as the MEAL team or department.

Those in charge of monitoring, such as project supervisors or MEAL department staff, should have a strong understanding of the health project's monitoring indicators, targets and means of verification.

Using monitoring tools

Monitoring tools come in various forms, ranging from simple paper-based checklists and record books to advanced smartphones or tablets with computing, information storage, and retrieval capabilities.

In recent times, health projects have shifted towards electronic devices that can quickly record and send a large amount of data from project sites directly to the main project office. The country office based PM or a MEAL colleague, can easily retrieve in real time the site data transmitted to them by the field monitors (supervisors) using their devices. The project office can then use their computers to compile the data from all the project sites, analyze it, and track the status of project activities. There are several apps and programs for data entry at the site level and for data analysis at a more central level. Computer programs can create charts, flowcharts, lists, tables, and maps, making it easier to understand trends, outliers, and patterns.

The PM must ensure that the monitoring tools, whether paper checklists or electronic devices, are available for those who will monitor the project tasks and sub-tasks. The paper checklist or the handheld devices used for monitoring must have the indicators, targets, and means of verification against each activity already printed or uploaded.

Visiting project sites and collecting data

The next step is for the monitors (supervisors) to visit the project sites and collect data on each activity, then recording these on their monitoring tools. See Image 9.1. The 'means of verification' that are listed in the DAP and in the monitoring tools will guide them to the correct source of information for gathering activity data. For example,

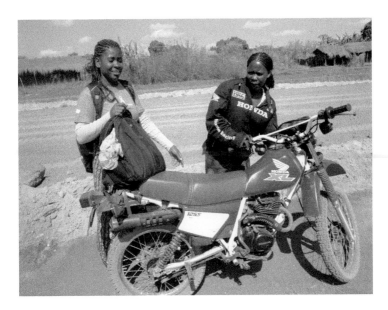

Image 9.1 Project supervisors preparing to visit sites for monitoring project activities in Mozambique

to monitor if vaccines are stored at the health centers at the correct temperature, the verification could be done using a logbook in these health centers.

The supervisors examine the logbook to ensure that the employees at the location where the vaccines are kept have correctly recorded the vaccine temperature in the logbook and indicated how often they have done so. A medication register can demonstrate whether a healthcare facility operated by the health project obtained and utilized medicines and materials for its patients as planned.

Again, the supervisor can verify an event such as a health education session for women by checking the session participant register. This is the register used for collecting signatures from all the session participants. The supervisor visits the location where this event takes place and records the findings from the register using a paper checklist or an electronic device. Supervisors often observe directly the evidence that an activity has been completed. See Image 9.2.

The project's total output target for every activity is divided among its various sites for each monitoring period. The target number will likely vary between sites from month to month or quarter to quarter based on

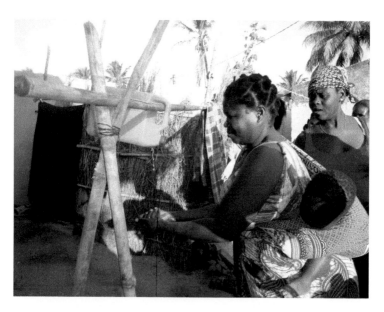

Image 9.2 The use of an installed 'Tippy Tap' observed by supervisor during monitoring visit in Mozambique

community size, needs, and seasonal and other factors. Supervisors who visit assigned sites should be aware of the target numbers for these sites, for example, installing a planned number of water pumps during the monitoring period for a certain site. This information (e.g. the planned number of water pumps) should be present in the paper checklist or the electronic device the supervisors use for data recording. Additionally, the PM or MEAL team colleague at the project (country) office will also have access to this planned target for each project site on their computers or checklists. They can determine the total number of pumps that were planned to be installed for the entire project by simply adding all the targets for all sites. After analyzing the data from the supervisors, it is easily determined if each site has met its planned pump installation target or if certain sites have fallen short. The monitoring tool provides space for notes, which the supervisors can use to record crucial information such as reasons for delays in pump installation or pump malfunctions, etc. This routine monitoring of project activities occurs monthly or quarterly, enabling the PM and health team to closely track progress at relatively short intervals.

Visiting project sites in person is highly beneficial for PMs as they can themselves observe the progress of project activities. Besides monitoring, such on-site visits also offer opportunities for coaching, mentoring, and problem-solving. The project team is motivated as they feel their contributions are valued and their concerns are heard by the PM, who is often based in the distant national capital. There should be detailed plans prepared for site visits for both supervisors and PMs. These plans should include the names of sites to be visited along with dates, times, objectives of the visit, and other relevant information. These details are important to include in project reports that the PM submits to senior management.

Table 9.1 gives a fictitious sample of a supervisory checklist used for monitoring of eight activities under two interventions in one village site.

A global health project may have multiple interventions (the sample checklist in Table 9.1 shows only two) with several tasks and sub-tasks. All these tasks and sub-tasks need routine monitoring. This comprehensive approach enables the PM to identify problems with specific sites or tasks that require attention.

In certain situations, such as security concerns or natural disasters, supervisors are prevented from physically visiting project sites. However, the staff members working at these sites can still utilize their electronic devices such as cell phones and tablets to send photos, video clips, or text messages to their supervisors to demonstrate the outputs of their activities. While this method may not provide complete information, the

Table 9.1 Sample monitoring checklist

Quarterly Monitoring checklist for Health Project
Anywhere District, Somewhere Land
Quarter ___1___   Project Site _____ Happy village _____
Supervisor/Monitor _____   Signature of supervisor/monitor _____
Date of visit _____

	Task No.	Task	Indicator	Means of verification	Target (Nos)	Task status (Nos)	Note
Intervention 1: Water & sanitation	1	Install handpumps	No. of handpumps installed	Site visit for counting handpumps	4	3	1 pump is delayed. Supply low.
	2	Instruct community members on maintenance of handpumps	No. of community members instructed in orientation session	Participants attendance register for orientation session	12	11	92%
	3	Invite Village Chief to attend handover ceremony	No. of Village Chiefs attending ceremony	Photos/video clips from handpump handover ceremony	2	2	100%
	4	Place posters in marketplace and at govt. health centers promoting use of water from handpumps	No. of posters placed in designated places	Village health workers' report and photos	7	9	UNICEF donated 2 extra posters to the project
	Task No.	Task	Indicator	Means of verification	Target (Nos)	Task status (Nos)	Note
Intervention 2: Child immunization	1	Give routine immunization to children under two years of age	No. of children vaccinated with all antigens	Immunization card shown by caregiver	96	73	76% covered. Flood caused many families to leave village
	2	Train Govt. HC staff on cold chain maintenance	No. of Govt. HC staff trained	Training report	6	2	33%. Govt. health dept. staff went on strike.
	3	Educate caregivers of children on child immunization	No. of caregivers received education	Participants attendance register	26	18	69%. Many left village due to flooding
	4	Donate vaccine carriers to govt. HCs	No. of vaccine carriers donated	HC equipment inventory record	4	4	100%

use of cell phones, tablets, and computers to transmit images, written reports, or voice recordings related to project activities are becoming increasingly popular and making great contributions to monitoring. This approach is commonly referred to as 'remote monitoring.'

During the Ebola outbreak in West Africa from 2014 to 2016 and more recently the COVID-19 pandemic, many countries were under lockdown, making it impossible for supervisors to travel to project sites. In these instances, supervisors relied on contact through cell phones, Skype, and Zoom to remotely communicate with their team members and monitor project outputs.

Conducting spot checks

Usually, those that monitor project activities and the PM prepare their individual monthly or quarterly calendars for visiting their sites. They let their site staff know in advance of the schedules of their visits. There are times, however, when the PM or a supervisor may want to conduct a random, unannounced 'spot check.' Chapter 5 gives more details on spot checks.

Analyzing monitoring data

Although project supervisors are typically responsible for on-site monitoring, it is the PM who utilizes the collected data to analyze the project's outputs. MEAL Team colleagues provide the PM with necessary support on the analysis. To effectively analyze project performance, the PM must receive monitoring data from all project sites each month or quarter in a timely manner.

Usually, the MEAL specialists create computer spreadsheets for the health project. These spreadsheets are designed to capture each site's outputs for each activity, for each monitoring period. By calculating the figures from all sites, computer programs can provide the total quantitative performance for each task and sub-task per site, per monitoring period, and for the entire project.

As a result, the PM has information on the project's overall performance as well as individual site performance for each monitoring period. This allows the PM to quickly identify any sites or activities that are falling behind and take necessary corrective actions in a timely manner.

The PM's reports on the project to senior managers become quite informative and useful when they include in it the project progress, over- or under-achievements, and also any corrective measures taken, along with the graphics generated from the computer program. Chapter 11 gives details on project reporting.

Utilizing monitoring data to improve health projects – a personal experience

Throughout this chapter, we explored the importance of monitoring, which enables the PM to track project progress and detect performance issues.

While managing a large-scale NGO-run global health project in Bangladesh early in my career, our project team closely collaborated with the MOH to support its EPI program. In this project, we implemented a monitoring and supervision model that played a pivotal role in enhancing the performance of government health workers responsible for immunizing children and women.

We developed checklists for monitoring the outputs from all of the project tasks to gather comprehensive information not only on whether a task was completed but also on its quality. Our POs analyzed the data collected by government supervisors who conducted monitoring visits to hundreds of immunization sites every month using the checklists. The project POs compiled and analyzed the information to identify trends and select a topic for each month's training, focusing on areas needing improvement.

On pay day each month, when the government workers responsible for administering vaccines (the CHWs) visited the district health offices to collect their pay, they also received a refresher training on the selected topic for that month. This 'monitoring → data analysis → training → monitoring' model continued throughout the project, ensuring ongoing performance improvement of the CHWs. The project model is depicted in Figure 9.1. I personally witnessed how

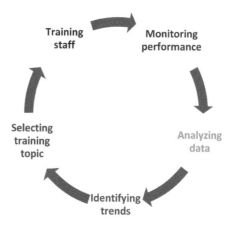

Figure 9.1 Project model showing the use of monitoring data

project monitoring can powerfully lead to continuous improvement in performance.

Key takeaways

- The PM employs monitoring of health projects to routinely track the progress of activities.
- Monitoring of projects requires the use of indicators, which are the yardsticks for measuring project outputs.
- For monitoring of health projects, the PM should focus mainly on output and input indicators. The *outcome* indicators are more useful for project *evaluations*.
- Besides indicators, the supervisors or monitors need targets and 'means of verification' to conduct monitoring of project activities.
- Paper-based checklists, smartphones, tablets, and computers are some tools that supervisors use for monitoring health projects.
- Monitoring often involves visits to the project sites, collecting data on each activity, and recording the data using the monitoring tools.
- The 'means of verification' selected during project planning (as in the DAP) guides supervisors to the source from where they can collect information about the outputs of tasks and sub-tasks.
- Remote monitoring takes place when physical visits by the supervisor is not feasible. Site staff can send photos, video clips, written reports or voice recordings to their supervisors using cell phones, computers and other devices.
- Spot checks are random unannounced visits made by monitoring staff at project sites.
- When data from monitoring is used to design staff training on an ongoing basis, it can contribute to continuous improvement of a health project.

Discussion questions

1. What can be an output indicator of a project that distributes mosquito bed nets to households? What can be a 'means of verification' for monitoring this output?
2. What would be an outcome indicator for this same activity?
3. What are the key items in the DAP that one needs for monitoring a project activity?

4. True or false questions: For each numbered statement in Table 9.2 write 'T' or 'F' to indicate 'True' or 'False' respectively.

Table 9.2 True or false questions

No.	Statements	T / F
1.	Monitoring of health projects assess the health of the community members.	
2.	Number of children that received polio vaccine in the previous month is a useful output indicator for project monitoring.	
3.	For verification of children that were vaccinated in the previous month the supervisors need to review the project proposal.	
4.	Not all sites in a multi-site health project can be expected to have an equal volume of target for a given activity.	
5.	Monitoring visits take place routinely every month or every quarter.	
6.	Remote monitoring takes place when supervisors arrive to assess project activities in a remote site.	

See correct answers on page 194.

Case study exercise

Imagine you are the PM of a project that operates in a mountainous region of an LMIC. An avalanche has completely blocked off the road to your project sites. Supervisors are unable to reach the sites and assess project activities. How can monitoring of site activities still take place?

See Author's suggestion on page 199–200.

10 Evaluating health projects

As my project management role for the global health project in Nagorno Karabakh was coming to an end, I decided to conduct an end-of-project evaluation, also known as a 'final evaluation.' However, there was disagreement within my organization's headquarters about whether such an evaluation was necessary for this project.

To address this, I posed some important questions to those who did not see the need for a final evaluation:

- How would we know if the project had produced the desired results if we didn't evaluate it?
- Even if the project had shown positive results, how would we know how to improve it for next time?
- And without an evaluation, how would our organization know if the project was worth replicating in this or other communities?

Ultimately, we agreed to proceed with the final evaluation of the project. Upon analyzing the data we gathered, we found:

- The project had exceeded nearly all its targets in all its interventions and activities.
- Some strategies could be improved for future projects.
- The communities we served and the local health administration we supported would benefit from a similar project in the future.

In our daily life, we analyze the value of our actions almost all the time. We research and find answers to our questions, discuss with others, evaluate feedback and findings we gather, and based on this information we make decisions on how to improve our efforts.

These informal assessments are generally adequate when the stakes are low. However, when large amounts of funding are involved or a significant number of people may be impacted by a project, the PM and the

DOI: 10.4324/9781003405245-11

implementing organization should invest in formal, visible, and scientific evaluation procedures.[1] Increasingly, funders and other stakeholders are requiring high quality evaluations of global health initiatives.

The evaluation of a project involves a systematic investigation of its merit, value, or significance. The purpose is to determine the project's efficiency and effectiveness and to make recommendations for improving its outcomes. This process includes collecting and analyzing data to assess the project's performance in achieving its objectives and its impact on the communities it serves, which includes both – benefits it accomplished and problems it has caused.

Evaluation provides answers to important questions such as whether the project can or should be replicated and why. It is also essential to identify any issues encountered during implementation. Evaluating a global health project allows the understanding and improvements of the health of the community it serves. The findings from the evaluation are valuable for learning, contributing to global health dialogue beyond the immediate project, and improving future global health efforts.

In the previous chapter, you learned that monitoring involves keeping track of the direct outputs of project tasks and sub-tasks. Evaluation, on the other hand, measures the *change* that the project brings about in the community – this is the project's *outcome.*

For instance, calculating the number of people who received the complete set of COVID-19 vaccines according to local protocol is monitoring the output of the project's vaccination activities. *Evaluating* the project's outcomes, on the other hand, involves calculating the *proportion* (percentage) of community members who did not contract the disease following the vaccination campaign.

Similarly, to properly assess the success of a project designed to improve maternal health in a community, one needs to consider more than just the number of women who attended educational sessions on safe delivery. That would be monitoring – the counting of immediate and direct output of a project task (the task being the organizing of health education sessions on safe delivery). Instead, evaluation calculates the proportion of women in the project area who gave birth at a health center. The ultimate goal of the project's education sessions on safe delivery is to bring about a positive *change* among pregnant women in the community - namely, increasing the number and proportion of women giving birth at health centers.

Types of project evaluations

The evaluations of global health projects are typically of three types – *baseline, midterm,* and *final evaluation* – based on when in the project's life the evaluation takes place.

The *baseline evaluation* takes place at the beginning of the project. It indicates what the health situation is in the project community before the project commences its interventions and activities. The baseline evaluation establishes the benchmark against which the PM will measure project achievements through subsequent evaluations.

The *mid-term evaluation*, as the term implies, occurs in the middle of a project's lifespan. It follows the same methodology as the baseline evaluation with the same indicators, questionnaire, and sampling of respondents. The mid-term evaluation reveals any changes that have occurred in the project communities up to that point. This allows the PM to make mid-course adjustments to project activities, objectives, or both if the mid-term evaluation indicates a need. This type of evaluation is also known as a 'mid-term review.'

Then, the *end-of-project* or *final evaluation* takes place when the project has either ended or is nearing completion. The final evaluation provides an assessment of the project's value and accomplishments. It is a thorough evaluation that examines whether the project was able to deliver what it had planned, the level of community participation, client satisfaction, changes in participant behavior, and changes in the community and environment. The final evaluation employs the same indicators as the previous two evaluations, allowing for comparison of results. Additionally, there are other indicators that help to answer the broader questions mentioned above.

The PM and their team may undertake *special evaluations* during various stages of the project cycle if deemed necessary. These may include repeat evaluations to confirm earlier findings, further examination of project aspects that were previously overlooked, or post-project evaluations to determine if community benefits have been sustained over time. Some global health projects might incorporate a research component. A special evaluation would be needed to study the research findings.

Standardized approaches are followed for all types of evaluations. Let us briefly go over each one.

Involving stakeholders

Members of the project community, particularly those in leadership roles, can provide significant value to project evaluations. Religious and political leaders, schoolteachers, and village elders can all offer their wisdom to make the evaluation more practical and representative.

In addition to community leaders, local government representatives, members of the business community, partner organizations, and funding agencies in the project area should be invited to participate in the evaluation process. Each stakeholder brings unique inputs and perspectives to the planning and execution of evaluation activities. A successful evaluation should

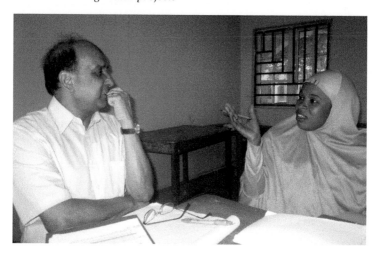

Image 10.1 Discussion with an FBO leader in northern Nigeria regarding project evaluation plans

consider the input and guidance of these stakeholders. It is important for them to feel ownership over the evaluation process, as the findings and learnings from the evaluation will impact them in various ways. Without their involvement in the planning stage, there may be resistance or disregard towards the evaluation. Engaging stakeholders in the process will likely lead to their approval and support, ensuring the evaluation runs smoothly. Image 10.1 shows the author and a local leader planning a final evaluation.

Developing a practical evaluation plan

The MEAL Team of the project implementing organization comprised of experts in evaluation, typically take the lead in designing the technical evaluations. The PM's role is to support this evaluation team by facilitating the evaluation activities. For the final evaluation, it may be beneficial to engage an external consultant or team of consultants from outside the implementing organization to act as an unbiased third party evaluator. With support from the PM and the project team, the evaluators will create a plan and schedule evaluation activities. This plan will include the team getting briefings on the project; reviewing project documents such as the project proposal, the DAP, and budget; and studying important communications, records, and materials both within and outside of the project to conduct a comprehensive evaluation. The MEAL staff or external consultant and their evaluation team will need to access these relevant documents and materials. The more the evaluator understands the health project, the better the quality of the evaluation. For example, they will need to carefully examine the DAP document to identify objectives, outcomes, outputs, activities, and indicators for measuring project performance, as well as sources to verify project activities and their outcomes, and any assumptions and risk factors that had been considered for project operations. See Chapter 3 for details on the DAP.

The plans for reviewing project documents, developing evaluation instruments such as questionnaires and checklists, visiting project sites to collect data, conducting meetings and discussions with key individuals and groups to collect their responses, analyzing the collected data, and finally disseminating the results of the evaluation with all concerned, will heavily involve the PM and the project team.

If the PM has a technical background, they might want to contribute directly to the evaluation process. But even if they are not technically oriented, they still facilitate the execution of the evaluation plan.

While leading a team of evaluators for a final evaluation of a reproductive health project in two large states of northern Nigeria I had an interesting experience. When I arrived in the capital, Abuja for the evaluation, one of the first things I did was to meet with the senior staff members of the project that had just been completed. The next step was for me and my team to travel to the project communities to collect evaluation data.

Then, following our visits to the project sites we met with the same project staff once again to go over with them my team's findings. This gave me and my team a chance to get more clarity on certain things about the project and receive valuable perspectives from these project staff on key issues. I was confident that we had reliable results not only because we gathered information from many different sources in the field, but we also consulted the project personnel after our field work on some findings that appeared confusing. And they helped clarify these issues.

The PM for the agency that oversaw this evaluation, had organized all our travels including the travels to and from Abuja for the two senior project staff who met with us two times, before and after data gathering. I was grateful to the PM for this type of forward thinking.

Collecting credible evidence

During project evaluations, evaluators gather information from various sources utilizing survey questionnaires, checklists, and observation guidelines. The sources include project participants, such as community members, as well as individuals who have directly or indirectly benefited from the project or were involved in its implementation. The latter group may include government health workers, community leaders, political or religious figures, and key project staff. The evaluation team may wish to group these individuals based on whether they provide quantitative data or qualitative information.

Quantitative data

In a simple population-based survey the evaluation team uses mathematical formula and other criteria to randomly select a sample of individuals (e.g. women of reproductive age; or mothers of children that are two years of age or younger) from the total population of the project community. This sample should be a good representation of the entire community where the project operated. The data collectors administer a survey questionnaire to each individual. See Image 10.2.

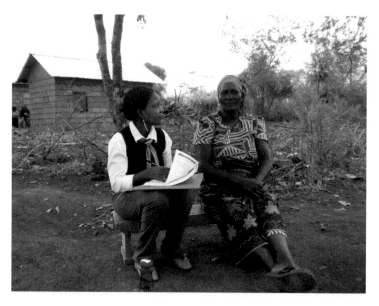

Image 10.2 Data collector using written questionnaires in an evaluation survey in Kenya

The survey is designed to quantify the answers given during individual interviews. For example, in a village, the data collectors may find a certain number of women respondents had taken two doses of tetanus toxoid vaccine during their most recent pregnancy. This data is analyzed and generalized to determine the vaccine coverage for all pregnant women in the entire community. Such an evaluation might also correlate vaccine coverage with the incidence of tetanus cases among pregnant women and newborns.

When all the answers have been collected and analyzed, a reliable snapshot of the community emerges. The sampling and the survey done in the proper way allow for the generalization of the findings to the entire project target area.

Qualitative data

When evaluating a project, simply relying on quantitative data is not enough to get a complete assessment. Evaluators also need to examine *quality* issues, which can indicate the project's value, its appropriateness, and whether it should continue or be replicated elsewhere. To thoroughly analyze these aspects, it is best to also consider *qualitative* data.

Qualitative evaluations go beyond just gathering numerical data. These also aim to uncover the underlying causes behind the figures. For instance, when it comes to assessing the prevalence of malaria among young children, a qualitative approach would not just look at how many malaria cases there were in the past year. It would also delve into the *reasons* why these children got infected with the disease. Was it because they did not use mosquito bed nets when sleeping? If not, what were the *reasons* behind this? Were the nets not available, or were they too expensive for most families?

During quantitative assessments, respondents who have benefited from a project are asked questions individually using structured questionnaires. In contrast, qualitative assessment typically involves interviewing individuals and groups using semi-structured qualitative questionnaires.

Key Informant Interviews (KIIs) take place with selected individuals who can provide valuable information on the project's functions, benefits, and deficiencies. Examples of KIIs include interviewing a nurse at a health center, a respected religious leader in the community, or a project staff member involved in project tasks.

Focus Group Discussions (FGDs) involve leading a discussion with a homogenous group of individuals, such as mothers, young school students, or farmers. The evaluators select group members based on specific criteria and facilitate the conversation to collect useful information about the project. FGDs are not interviews, but rather a participatory

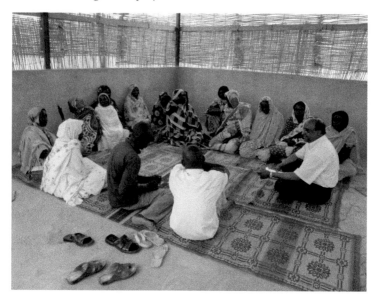

Image 10.3 An FGD session with village women in Chad

group discussion where everyone can share their information and opinions. See Image 10.3.

When evaluators use both quantitative and qualitative methodologies in an evaluation, they adopt a *mixed methodology*. Although quite involved, this approach provides a fuller assessment of a project.

Analyzing and synthesizing collected information

After data collection, the evaluation team proceeds with data cleaning to ensure that any errors made while recording the data are corrected. This meticulous process involves addressing questions in the questionnaire that are left blank or shows unclear responses, allowing evaluators to use only meaningful data.

The next step involves *analyzing* and *synthesizing* different data to arrive at a larger result, which is the evaluation's findings. The evaluators make interpretations based on the analyzed and synthesized data. For example, if 95 percent of the respondents visited the health center for ANC services at least twice during their recent pregnancy, the evaluators would want to know what this means from the stakeholders' point of view. They would consider other results, such as those from the FGD where the respondents may have discussed how they spent a significant amount of money on bus tickets to visit the distant health center, which affected their family finances. Will the 95 percent be interpreted as success, or will the interpretation need to consider the financial burden the community members had to carry? The evaluators grapple with these and similar questions before making conclusions about the project's success and worth.

To analyze quantitative data, the evaluators use statistical methods to describe, summarize, and compare numerical data.[2] They can calculate and compare frequencies, percentages, ratios, mean, median, and mode with the cleaned field data using computer software programs. An experienced data analyst can use such programs to draw accurate conclusions about the data.

> Many years ago, during a global health project evaluation in rural Mariupol, Ukraine, I was introduced to the Kobo ToolBox[3] by a local member of the organization's MEAL team. This free, open-source data collection and management software was developed by Kobo in partnership with UN agencies, the Harvard Humanitarian Initiative, and nonprofit organizations, specifically for use in challenging humanitarian settings. It has since become one of the most popular data handling software, used by over 14,000 organizations worldwide.
>
> We used Kobo ToolBox to create full questionnaires, collect survey data from the field, share data among team members in real-time, perform data analysis, and generate reports. Multiple individuals, both in Ukraine and outside of the country, simultaneously used the software to track data entry and analysis online. I continued to collaborate with the local team on this data management work using Kobo Toolbox even after returning to my office in the U.S. from Ukraine.

There are many software programs that can collect and analyze *qualitative* data. These online tools are collaborative and can assist the evaluation team in staying organized and competently analyze the data. One such software is 'ATLAS.ti,' which has been used by evaluators for some time. Additionally, there are businesses that offer off-the-shelf and customized software with technical support to help set up and run qualitative data collection and analysis for projects. The MEAL colleagues may be familiar with many of them.

Making justifiable conclusions

To confidently use the evaluation results, the evaluation team and the project staff need to carefully consider the analyzed data from various stakeholders' perspectives before reaching conclusions. All stakeholders must agree that the conclusions reached are well-substantiated and justified.[4]

The conclusions will focus on the project's significance, value, or merit. Different stakeholders may have varying conclusions and judgments about a project. For example, an increase in the COVID-19 vaccination rate from ten percent to 55 percent in one year resulting from project efforts may seem like a great achievement to the PM and the project team. However, community leaders may view the same results and conclude that a 55 percent coverage rate is not impressive enough because many people in the community still contracted the disease or even passed away during that same period.

This example illustrates how different stakeholders may use different standards to make judgments about project success. Therefore, it is critical to find an agreement among all key stakeholders about the appropriate standards to use for making justifiable conclusions concerning the project.

Using the evaluation results and recommendations

When evaluating a health project, one must recognize that it serves a practical purpose beyond simply satisfying the demands of funding agencies or management. In fact, evaluations have important practical functions.

A baseline evaluation establishes a reference point at the outset of project implementation, the findings from which are compared to those of subsequent evaluations. The recommendations provided through this baseline evaluation can help with developing or modifying project design.

A midterm evaluation offers an opportunity to correct project plans or performance, based on the evaluation's recommendations. This could involve revising project objectives and targets or adjusting project tasks and sub-tasks.

A final evaluation determines the project's value and success by comparing its achievements to its intended objectives and outcomes. If successful, the evaluation may recommend continuing the health project in the same or an expanded geographical area. These findings may also justify replicating the project in another location, with either the same or modified project objectives, outcomes, and outputs.

Sharing the results

After completing an evaluation, the PM shares the results with relevant stakeholders in a transparent and unbiased manner. There are various ways to disseminate the findings, such as print formats, slide presentations, news releases, press conferences, radio and television coverage, and public meetings, email listservs, and web-based dissemination. This authentic communication with relevant stakeholders will help garner support for the project.[5]

Sharing the evaluation results with the project team members is also essential. It will help them understand the project goals and objectives better, see the results of their efforts, and improve teamwork. It allows them to see their project activities from a different angle, reinforcing or questioning assumptions that link these activities to the anticipated effects. The sharing of the evaluation results also leads the team to develop a collective vision for the project.

One crucial step is to share the evaluation findings and recommendations with the community members where the project is operating. Many of them participated in the evaluation surveys, KIIs, and FGDs, and they are directly impacted by the health project and deserve to be informed in a way that they can understand. This effort will not only be appreciated by them, but also encourage them to cooperate with the project team members more eagerly, leading to a meaningful project partnership.

Supporting the evaluation activities

Certain key activities for which the evaluators need support from the PM and their team include:

Reviewing of documents

To facilitate the evaluation process, evaluators require printed and electronic copies of all pertinent project documents, as listed earlier. Therefore, the PM and team should provide these materials to the evaluators at the start of the evaluation process ensuring there is sufficient time for them to analyze these materials.

Developing evaluation tools

The preparation for evaluation involves creating, testing, and producing survey questionnaires, checklists, and guidelines for KIIs and FGDs. The PM makes sure that the evaluators receive logistical assistance from the project team in designing the tools and get feedback on them.

Selecting and training data collectors

The evaluators require skilled individuals who can be trained to gather information from the communities using data collection tools. Ideally, the data collectors should come from the project communities. The project team assists in identifying and selecting data collectors and facilitates their training.

Traveling to project sites

The project staff is responsible for arranging travel for the evaluation team so they can easily visit the project communities and move around from one project site to another for collecting data. The project also assists with finding suitable accommodation for the evaluation team.

Collecting data from project communities

Those that are responsible for evaluating the project visit specific project sites to gather both quantitative and qualitative data. During travel between communities, the evaluators rely on the PM and their team to ensure safe transportation. Additionally, they require assistance in establishing contacts with government officials, community leaders, and villagers to set up interviews and discussions. The project team members are familiar with these individuals and assist in facilitating these interactions. If necessary, the project team recruits translators.

Synthesizing collected data and preparing evaluation report

The next step involves systematically transcribing and organizing the data and notes collected from the interactions in the community. The evaluation report is then consolidated, drafted, and finalized. At this stage, a significant amount of photocopying, storing, and sharing takes place. The evaluators need help with these activities from the PM and the project team.

Disseminating the evaluation report

The next step involves sharing the final evaluation report with the stakeholders. This may involve presentations and meetings. The PM, along with the project team, can strategically play an important role in disseminating the report.

> Earlier in the chapter, I mentioned leading an evaluation in northern Nigeria. The final task of the evaluation process was for me to write a 200-page report. The report included detailed information regarding the design, activities, findings, recommendations, and other aspects related to this significant undertaking.
>
> For sharing the report widely, the donor agency made it available online at the Development Experience Clearinghouse, the largest online resource library for USAID-funded technical and project materials.[6] Widespread dissemination of the evaluation report was quite important to them.

Key takeaways

- Evaluating a project involves a systematic investigation into its merit, value, and significance.
- This involves measuring the *outcomes* generated by the project, which are the changes it brings about in the community as a result of its activities.
- Depending on the stage of the project, there may be a baseline, mid-term, and final evaluation, with additional assessments sometimes needed in special situations.
- To ensure a thorough evaluation, it is standard practice to involve stakeholders, develop an evaluation plan, collect evidence (through data, information, and observations), analyze, and synthesize the data, draw evidence-based conclusions, make practical use of the evaluation results and recommendations, and share the results with all relevant parties.
- Usually, the MEAL colleagues or external consultants conduct evaluations. The PM and the health project team facilitate all the activities performed by the evaluators.

Discussion questions

1. How does project evaluation differ from project monitoring?
2. What are the standard approaches common to baseline, mid-term, and final evaluations?
3. Give three similarities and differences between quantitative and qualitative evaluations.
4. Who should receive the evaluation results and why?
5. True or false questions: For each numbered statement in Table 10.1 write 'T' or 'F' to indicate 'True' or 'False' respectively.

Table 10.1 True or false questions

No.	Statements	T/F
1.	Involving all the relevant stakeholders in project evaluation is beneficial.	
2.	Monitoring and evaluation both measure project *outputs*.	
3.	Evaluation gives a monthly picture of the progress that a project is making.	
4.	FGDs are a type of qualitative evaluation.	
5.	Baseline evaluation does not determine the value of a project.	
6.	Evaluation reports should not be shared with community members as they do not understand it.	

See correct answers on page 194.

Case study exercise

As the PM for a refugee health project at the Rohingya refugee camp in Cox's Bazar, Bangladesh, you receive a visit from the MEAL staff based at your organization's overseas headquarters. They are here to conduct a baseline evaluation of the project and require data collectors and supervisors. How can you and your team provide support to the MEAL colleagues with this particular need?

See Author's suggestion on page 200–201.

Notes

1 Milstein, B. and Wetterhall, S., "A Framework for Program Evaluation." *KU Center for Community Health and Development. CDC Evaluation Working Group: University of Kansas, Community Tool Box*. Last modified 2022, https://ctb.ku.edu/en/table-of-contents/evaluate/evaluation/framework-for-evaluation/main
2 "Analyzing Quantitative Data for Evaluation. Evaluation Briefs. No. 20," last updated August 2018, www.cdc.gov/ healthyyouth/evaluation/index. htm.
3 For more information on the Kobo ToolBox software program, please visit www.kobotoolbox.org/
4 Milstein, B. and Wetterhall, S., "A Framework."
5 "Evaluation Briefs No. 9: Disseminating Program Achievements and Evaluation Findings to Garner Support," last modified August 2018, accessed March 14, 2023, www.cdc.gov/healthyyouth/evaluation/pdf/ brief9.pdf
6 For downloading the report one can use the link https://pdf.usaid.gov/pdf_docs/PA00JP52.pdf

References

Milstein, B. and Wetterhall, S., "A Framework for Program Evaluation." *KU Center for Community Health and Development. CDC Evaluation Working Group: University of Kansas, Community Toolbox*. Last modified 2022. https://ctb.ku.edu/en/table-of-contents/evaluate/evaluation/framework-for-evaluation/main

"Evaluation Briefs No. 9: Disseminating Program Achievements and Evaluation Findings to Garner Support." Last modified August 2018. www.cdc.gov/ healthyyouth/evaluation/pdf/ brief9.pdf

"Evaluation Briefs No. 20: Analyzing Quantitative Data for Evaluation." Last updated August 2018. www.cdc.gov/healthyyouth/evaluation/index.htm

The Mitchell Group, Inc., "The Leadership Development for Family Planning / Reproductive Health for Political Office Holders, Traditional and Religious Leaders Project." USAID/Nigeria's Monitoring and Evaluation Project II. Last modified 2014. https://pdf.usaid.gov/pdf_docs/PA00JP52.pdf

11 Reporting on project activities

During field visits to several countries, I had often said to PMs and their teammates, "*Doing good work in a health project is half the job done. The other half is to tell the world about the good work that you've done.*" I'd like to begin this chapter by sharing that same advice with you as you prepare to manage global health projects.

In the previous chapters, we covered the key responsibilities that the PM and their team carry out for implementing global health projects. Now, we will focus on how to *report* on these activities and the project's progress. This chapter will explore the essential elements of project reporting, including the purpose of project reports, the different types of reports, and the necessary steps and structure for writing them. But first, let us clarify what project reports actually are.

Project reports are an essential project management tool. By developing these reports and referring to past reports the PM and their project teams can gauge their project's implementation progress and fund status, identify problem areas that require urgent attention, and adjust their activities to accomplish the project's objectives on time. Also, project reports act as a useful record of decisions and actions taken throughout the project's lifecycle. Thus, these different types of reports contribute significantly to managing projects.

Besides functioning as a project management instrument for the PM, a global health project report serves as the primary tool for stakeholders and end users to understand the current status of a project.[1] Creating well-written project reports can be crucial in gaining support from the public, government, and funding agencies. While multiple team members may contribute to drafting the report, the PM is responsible for reviewing, finalizing, and submitting it.

In a typical global health project, the MOH might require information on the number of COVID-19 patients tested and confirmed positive at project health centers during a specific reporting period, such

DOI: 10.4324/9781003405245-12

as the past quarter. The funding agency may request financial information from the PM regarding the project's expenses. And the senior management at the organizational headquarters expects the PM to provide monthly or quarterly reports outlining the project's performance and financial status. The PM's report not only assists in tracking project progress but also contributes to the creation of annual reports and updating websites or social media content for the entire organization, whether it is the MOH or an NGO.

Types of project reports

Throughout the course of a global health project, the PM may create and submit various types of reports to stakeholders. Here we consider six types of project reports: progress reports, annual reports, trip reports, monitoring and evaluation reports, donor reports, and project termination reports. Although the PM is not solely responsible for drafting all these reports, they typically oversee the process and delegate certain report developing tasks to team members and external consultants. For instance, the final evaluation report is usually a collaborative effort involving multiple contributors under the PM's supervision.

Progress reports

Creating and submitting routine project progress reports to stakeholders is a critical responsibility of the PM. These reports, which can be monthly or quarterly, give updates on the health project's performance to senior management, funding agencies, MOH counterparts, and team members.

The progress report gives a useful reflection of the status of ongoing project activities. It allows recipients to easily identify which tasks are on track, partially done, or not yet completed. For example, senior management may need to know about the completion of a polio vaccination campaign that was scheduled for the previous quarter. If the task is still unfinished, the report should explain the reasons behind the delay and provide a plan for completing it in a timely manner. In addition, the progress report provides important information about obstacles, challenges, and risks that could affect project outcomes.

When preparing a progress report, the PM presents key information clearly to the recipients. This includes:

- Assessment of the project's progress by comparing it to the DAP (see Chapter 3), which outlines each task and sub-task. This comparison is done with data collected through routine project monitoring, which is discussed in Chapter 9.

- List of planned activities for the upcoming reporting period, which may be a quarter or a month.
- Analysis of the project's financial status, such as the BvA variance for each line item, and indicating any overspending or underspending that occurred (see Chapter 8).
- Discussion of any risks that the project has faced or may face in the future, and outlining any steps taken or needed to address them.
- Review of any other significant factors that may have impacted the project's goals and implementation or could do so in the future.

The MOH and NGOs usually have their standardized reporting formats for all projects they operate. When submitting a progress report, the PM follows this standardized format. Some organizations may require two separate reports, a *technical* report, and a *financial* report, for the same reporting period, while others prefer a combined report that includes both sections.

In a combined report, the technical section typically includes a narrative sub-section and a sub-section with quantitative information on project outputs. The financial section mainly provides budget and expenditure figures, but also includes a narrative section that explains these figures, particularly if there is a variance between budget and expenditure. Figure 11.1 outlines the format of a combined technical and financial progress report.

- General information. The progress report begins with a general section.

  - Name and place of the project.
  - Title or heading of the report. Tells the audience at the very beginning if this is a quarterly or monthly progress report.
  - Name and title of the person writing the report. Usually, it is the PM that writes or reviews, finalizes, and submits progress reports.
  - Date. This is the date of report submission. Dating the reports helps the recipients to compare them and evaluate the progress the project has made over time.

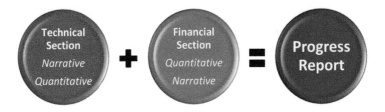

Figure 11.1 Progress report structure

- Technical section. Following are the elements of the technical narrative:

  - Summary of the project. This section should begin with a brief synopsis of the project objectives. This tells the recipients what the project is all about.
  - Discussion of tasks and sub-tasks. Next, the PM provides detailed information on each task and sub-task. These can be for instance, the distribution of malaria bed nets, installation of hand pumps for clean water, and training of CHWs on Integrated Community Case Management. Here the report describes how many of these activities were completed, which sites were most successful and why, any challenges encountered during implementation, and other pertinent details. This narrative part is an essential and extensive element of the technical report.
  - Quantitative report on tasks. The project report should also include a *quantitative* sub-section where numerical values demonstrate progress against planned targets. This is in addition to, and normally follows the narrative discussion of project achievements covered under the preceding bullet point.

    Some organizations require the submission of these numerical values from each project site or district. Others may need only the aggregate value (compiled from the numbers of each site or district), which reflects the entire project's performance. In either case, the PM will need to have quantitative information from all the project sites, particularly for tracking each site and following up with them as needed. A table with rows and columns is an effective way to present the project performance in a quantitative manner as illustrated in Table 11.1. This illustrative table is a sample of a quantitative sub-section of the technical part of the report.

Table 11.1 Quantitative reporting of project activities, their targets, achievements, and deviations

Activity number	Activity	Target	Achievement	Deviation
4.3.	No. of malaria bed nets distributed	500	350	−150
4.4.	No. of hand pumps installed	60	63	+3
4.5.	No. of CHWs trained	400	120	−280
4.6.				
4.7.				

Brief reason for deviation:
4.3. Rain and mudslide prevented distribution. Plan is made to increase distribution next quarter to achieve target.
4.4. Three additional pumps were installed at the request of the village leaders. Vendor supplied these free of cost.
4.5. A large number of CHWs went on strike demanding pay increase from the MOH. Following resolution of this issue the project will train the remaining CHWs that missed the training.

There is space (a column) in this table to record any deviation, which is the difference between the planned numerical target and the achievement value for each activity.

The format usually has a space just below (or next to) these numerical entries where one can write the reasons for any deviation that may have occurred.

- Plans for next quarter. This element of the report highlights the key project activities planned for the following reporting period (e.g., quarter). This gives continuity to the reports.

- Financial section. The progress report has so far focused on the technical achievements of the project during the reporting period. Now, the report addresses the *financial* status of the project.

To prepare this section of the report, the PM relies on the expertise of the finance department colleagues. They are experienced in financial analysis and report generation. The project team may have a finance colleague working within the project, or the country office where the PM is based may have a small finance unit. The country office's finance unit normally has direct links with the organization's finance department located at the headquarters or a regional office.

The finance colleagues need reliable financial data to help with financial analysis and report generation. Thus, the PM and their team members need to provide the finance colleagues with all the information on the expenditure incurred for each budget line item. Every member of the project team submits expense receipts and related paperwork throughout the project life, so that these are available to the finance staff when needed.

The finance staff already has the project's budget and budget-related documents, which they will use to compare with project expenditure for each line item. They will likely use financial software packages to generate a draft financial report for the PM's review to help track the BvA variance accurately. The role of the finance department in supporting the project is discussed in Chapter 8.

When it comes to comparing planned targets with actual expenses, financial reporting is similar to the technical narrative reporting. The financial section also includes a shorter narrative part that analyzes and explains key expenditures. If there are significant deviations between the budget and actual expenses for specific line items, the narrative part will provide explanations. The organization's finance department and/or funding agency sets a percentage threshold for these deviations. Deviations that go beyond this threshold require explanations. The department uses a standard template to report on project finances, which helps the organization track expenses across all its projects.

- Special notes. The progress report includes additional details about the project. For instance, any challenges the project team encountered during operations, innovative strategies implemented and their outcomes, and anticipated risks that may arise in the future, along with the measures needed to mitigate them. Additionally, the report should highlight the impact of the assumptions that were made during the planning stage on the project, especially if they proved to be correct. Lastly, any unexpected expenses should be explained, including the amount spent.
- Signature and date. The report normally ends with the PM's signature and date. This signifies to the recipients that the PM has thoroughly reviewed the document and is in agreement with its contents.

Annual reports

The annual report is a comprehensive overview of the activities the project undertook throughout a year of implementation. It is more voluminous than the monthly or quarterly progress reports as it covers a longer period of time. Like a progress report, the main body of an annual report contains technical and financial sections. However, it evaluates the project's performance for the entire year, offering a thorough analysis of the technical and financial performance for each quarter. The presentation format for the technical and financial sections of the annual report is similar to that of the progress report, which we discussed above. Additionally, the annual report usually includes an Executive Summary section and a Conclusion.

- Executive Summary. The annual report usually starts with an executive summary that briefly outlines the report's content. This summary should give a concise overview of the report, allowing the reader to understand its key points without having to go through the entire document.
- Conclusion. The annual report ends with a brief overview of the main components discussed in the document. It is also a good idea to outline in this concluding sub-section the upcoming plans for the project in the next reporting period and any action that readers may need to take after reading the report.
- Signature and date. As in the case of progress reports the PM also signs and dates the annual report.

Trip reports

The PM frequently visits health project sites to supervise project activities, interact with site managers and their teams, conduct training sessions or OJT, hold meetings with local government officials (especially MOH staff), and meet with community leaders and members in VDCs and VHCs. The PM writes a trip report after each field trip, which is usually required by most implementing agencies. The report should contain only essential information regarding the site visit and need not be excessively detailed. PMs usually have a checklist to ensure they cover all key activities during their site visits.

A typical trip report for a site monitoring visit may include:

- Name of project and name of project site visited.
- Date and Time of the site visit.
- Name of project's site manager or key team member based at the site.
- List of key individuals especially outside the project that the PM met during the visit.
- Project background. A brief description of what the project goal and objectives are, and any special activities that are taking place at the visited site.
- Objective of the visit. The purpose of the trip, whether a routine visit, or visit for a special occasion, such as site monitoring or training.
- Findings. Key things the PM observed at the site, for instance, children received their routine vaccinations, health education sessions took place, the need to improve cleanliness in the patient waiting area, or the need to update vaccination records in the logbook.
- Actions. Any actions the PM has taken, for instance, holding a teaching session for the site team members.
- Recommendations. Anything the PM may have recommended, such as reorganizing the dispensary of the project health center.
- Follow up. List of items that should be followed up during subsequent visits.
- Conclusion. Concluding remarks highlighting critical areas of the report.
- Photos. It is quite useful to incorporate field photos into the written report. As the saying goes, *"a picture is worth a thousand words,"* and photos can effectively showcase project activities. The photos are well received if they demonstrate actions or items of interest pertaining to project activities.
- Signature, name, title, and date. These are important elements to include at the end of the report. These ensure that one can reach out to the author of the report if there is any question, or if clarifications are needed in connection with the visit.

In addition to providing information about site visits, trip reports also serve as a management tool by allowing for comparisons of improvements and changes at project sites. Besides the PM there are others in the team that will make regular site visits, such as those with supervisory roles. They too should write their individual trip reports and submit to you, so that as the PM you can view their perspectives on site activities of the entire project.

Evaluation reports

These specialized reports detail the evaluation activities of the health project. Typically, the organization's MEAL colleagues are responsible for creating these reports after completing the project evaluation. In some cases, external technical consultants may be brought on board, especially for conducting the final evaluation of the health project as mentioned in the previous chapter. In that case, these external consultants usually write the evaluation reports.

Although the PM is not directly responsible for writing these reports, they review the draft reports and offer suggestions for improvement. After these reports are reviewed and finalized the PM submits these to the senior level staff at the country office (Country Director/Chief of Party), the regional office, or the headquarters of their organization.

Donor reports

From time to time, the agency providing funding to the project may ask for specific reports regarding how the awarded funds are being utilized. These financial reports can be requested on an ad hoc basis, or the donor agency may establish a regular schedule for their submission.

Normally though, the donor organization does not directly ask the PM for such reports. Instead, the implementing organization's headquarters establishes a reporting process with project donors. Usually, any report that the PM and their team prepare for the donor is first submitted to the implementing organization's regional office or headquarters for careful review. There are certain expenses (e.g., overhead costs) at the regional or headquarters level, which are added to the project costs and included in the donor report. The regional office or headquarters will thus submit a more complete financial report to the donor. Donor agencies usually accept progress and annual reports from the implementing organization's headquarters, which typically include financial sections.

Project termination report

A global health project may end for various reasons. It could terminate as scheduled following the completion of its activities, or during implementation due to unforeseen crises such as violent conflicts or security threats. Termination may also result from the donor agency halting funding, or changes in government or organizational policies. Regardless of the reason, the PM must provide an official project closure report to inform stakeholders about the termination's cause, end date, pending activities, and plans to withdraw assets from project areas.

The project termination report must include total expenditures, BvA variance, project implementation details including its achievements, variances related to activity schedule, changes in staffing, and other relevant information. A 'Lessons Learned' section should also be included to briefly discuss what the team learned during the life of the project and what could be applied to future projects. This section should also highlight any special occasion or difficulties that occurred during project implementation.

Suggestions on writing project reports

- When creating reports, it is vital to keep them concise and straightforward. Providing excessive information not only takes up the report writer's time but also that of the stakeholders. To ensure that the reports are well received, it is best to keep them focused and to-the-point. This applies to all types of reports, from progress updates to donor reports and annual reports.
- It is also critical to pay attention to page limits, which are often prescribed for reports. This means that you will need to organize and present a large volume of information in a concise manner.
- It is recommended that the PM keep technical language as simple as possible, as not all recipients will be familiar with the technical jargon and acronyms used in project operations.
- To make the reports more engaging and easier to understand, consider using visual elements such as images, graphs, charts, diagrams, and tables. These can help to express information concisely and add variety to the reports. When using visuals, it is important to keep them simple and not overly complicated.
- During field trips and office events, one should take photos and collect materials that can be presented and discussed in the reports. Statements from community leaders, government and donor representatives, and members of the community can be used in reports to make important points. Additionally, human interest stories from those who have benefited from the project can provide powerful testimonies in the reports.
- If there are actions the PM expects the recipients to take after reading the report, they should clearly state them. For example, if one needs approval for a project activity or require increased resources, this should be highlighted in the relevant report.
- Before submitting a report, one must be sure to review, edit, and proofread it. The initial draft can always be improved, and sensitive statements

and information may need to be re-phrased or removed. Language, punctuation, and grammar may also require correction. Additionally, making reports concise and enjoyable to read can be beneficial.

- When submitting a report, you must always be honest and transparent. Stakeholders appreciate openness, even if the project has overspent its budget or has lagged behind in reaching certain milestones. The quicker they learn about any difficulties, the sooner they can help to get the project back on track.
- It is also important to anticipate questions that may arise following the report's submission, and to prepare well to answer them. Finally, you need to follow the organization's protocol for report submission. And, of course, you must always submit reports on time and avoid delays.

Key takeaways

- Project reports are an essential project management tool. These reports help to see if the project is on track. The PM can also use these reports to monitor project costs, possible risks, as well as the implementation of project activities.
- While these reports may be drafted by multiple team members, external consultants, and others, the PM is responsible for reviewing, finalizing, and submitting them.
- There may be different types of project reports, but the most important ones are the progress reports, annual reports, trip reports, monitoring and evaluation reports, donor reports, and project termination reports.
- The progress report is the most critical because it helps recipients understand which activities are on schedule, and which ones have not been completed. It includes both a technical and financial section. The financial section gives BvA variance for each line item in the budget plan.
- A progress report also includes a list of the activities that are planned for the *following* reporting period (e.g., quarter or month).
- It is quite important to discuss in the progress and annual reports the risks the project faced during the reporting period, how these were mitigated, and how these will be addressed in the future.
- For writing the financial section in the progress report and the annual report the PM will likely need support from the implementing organization's finance department. So, it is critical to ensure the expense receipts and related paperwork are in order and available for the finance staff when they need them.
- Incorporating field photos, charts, diagrams, and tables as well as human interest stories can make the reports more engaging and persuasive.
- The organization's MEAL staff can help with developing the project's monitoring and evaluation reports.

- When the project closes the PM should submit an official project termination report, giving to the stakeholders important information on project activities, closure date, any unexpected cause for project closure, and plans for the withdrawal of project assets from the project areas.
- Including a 'Lessons Learned' section in the project termination report is quite helpful. This section allows the PM to share with the recipients the valuable experiences gained by the project team throughout the project life.
- For improving report writing skills, one ought to consider these helpful suggestions: keeping reports concise; avoiding technical jargon; using visual elements; carefully reviewing, editing, and proofreading the reports; making reports honest and open; and following the implementation organization's reporting procedures.

Discussion questions

1. In addition to giving project related information to the stakeholders how else can project reports serve as project management tools?
2. Would you include in your report any incomplete activity or over expenditure in your project? Why or why not?
3. Why is it important to organize and submit in a timely manner the receipts and related documents for project costs?
4. Table 11.2 contains six numbered items covered in this chapter, with short descriptions in the right column. However, these descriptions are not arranged in the correct order and do not match the items on the left. Match each numbered item to its description on the right and correctly write the corresponding letter of the description in the middle column.

Table 11.2 Multiple choice questions

Match the following with the answers in the last column	Insert letter of the correct answer	Answer
1. Progress and annual reports.		A. Help make the reports persuasive and easily understood.
2. Trip reports.		B. Rely on expense receipts and related documents.
3. Evaluation reports.		C. Includes financial status of the project.
4. Visual elements.		D. Must be clearly explained in the progress and annual reports.
5. Finance department staff of the organization.		E. Usually, the MEAL colleagues help write these reports.
6. Budget vs. actual variance.		F. Give information about project site visits.

See correct answers on page 194.

Case study exercise

As the newly appointed PM for a complex health project in an LMIC, you are required to submit a project progress report to the Country Director at the end of each quarter. What steps can you take to ensure timely submission of these reports?

See Author's suggestion on page 201.

Note

1 Zeshan Naz, "Project Report: Objectives, Types, Use Cases, Templates," *Knowledgehut upGrad* (blog), April 19, 2023, www.knowledgehut.com/blog/project-management/project-report

Reference

Naz, Zeshan. 2023. "Project Report: Objectives, Types, Use Cases, Templates." *Knowledgehut upGrad* (blog). April 19. www.knowledgehut.com/blog/project-management/project-report

12 Some final thoughts

Congratulations on finishing the preceding chapters of this book! Hopefully, you have learned many essential lessons in the foregoing pages, from the basics of managing global health projects to closing projects and writing project reports. At this point, you may feel your learning journey is complete, but that is not true. The real journey has only just begun!

> When I finished my university course in global health, I thought I knew everything I needed to know about managing, advising, and directing global health projects. However, I quickly realized that practical experience is just as important as academic knowledge. Over three decades, I gained valuable hands-on expertise by traveling to and working in various LMICs around the world.

You will also need to add to your academic knowledge necessary practical proficiencies that will help you to effectively lead your project team and make your global health projects successful.

Coupled with the technical skills and practical proficiencies, you will want to develop *leadership* attributes that will place you in higher demand as a PM, providing a solid foundation that will enable you to adapt to the continually changing dynamics of global health projects.

Leadership attributes

In these final few pages of the book, let me highlight a few key leadership areas where a PM must *grow* in the real world of managing global health projects and *transform* into a successful organizational leader. These are different from the management functions you have read about thus far in this book. These are leadership qualities that will help in that growth and transformation. These qualities discussed here are fundamental building blocks that PMs cultivate in themselves as they gain

DOI: 10.4324/9781003405245-13

knowledge, experience, and wisdom to become strong, effective leaders in their organizations.

Beginning with the end in mind

Like most people, you also want to succeed in your career. You are studying hard and will apply your education in the practical field to eventually become a successful PM and leader in your organization. How does success look to you? How do you envision yourself to be when you have emerged as an effective leader of your team and in your organization? When you start your career, begin with that end picture in your mind. Develop specific goals even as you take your first step in managing your project team. A short-term goal can be to successfully manage a global health project that brings better health and well-being to a community in an LMIC. But a longer-term goal could be to become a mature advisor or a senior instructor in your organization, helping other relatively inexperienced PMs and their teams in multiple LMICs to develop their health project management skills and become successful in their career.

> Toward the end of an active career, this was my role – to work in the organizational headquarters, travel to many LMICs, help numerous teams and their PMs to run their global health projects well, and support them in developing new projects with innovative strategies.

> John Quincy Adams, the sixth president of the United States once said, *"If your actions inspire others to dream more, learn more, do more and become more, you are a leader."* Would you want to become such a leader at the end of your global health career? Then that is your end goal, and that is what you would want to prepare for even as you complete your study program and embark on your project management journey. You start your journey by leading your own health project team, but you go on to eventually contributing to the growth of many others. Study how influential leaders have made their mark in history. Follow the strategies they have used in their travel along their career path.

Building a strategic mindset

Successful PMs do not simply utilize their technical management skills. They look to the future and adopt a strategic view for directing their projects and aligning them to their organization's strategies. Understanding how the post-pandemic world since 2020 is influencing global health projects along with other types of projects is crucial. Today, complex internal and external factors can quickly negatively impact all projects.

For instance, in an uncontrolled disease outbreak, legal restrictions, remote project management, cultural issues, and significant resource constraints and delays have become a reality. PMs that quickly strategize to cope with and mitigate the effects of these unanticipated obstacles can become successful leaders in their organizations. Developing a mindset for facing and dealing with unexpected practicalities will be an important asset for you.

Motivating others

Project success hinges upon the stakeholders' cooperation, respect, and motivation, especially the sponsors or donors that fund and support your global health project. It is relatively easy to influence your team members; however, motivating the communities in the LMICs, funding agencies, MOH officials over whom you may have little or no direct influence is more difficult but paramount to project success. They can contribute to the success or failure of your health project.

You will need to motivate the community leaders, so they become organized into community health committees, taking ownership of the health activities that the project staff and volunteers conduct in their localities. You may need to convince the donors that an innovative approach you wish to introduce in your health project will indeed produce desired results. The MOH may require documentation from you showing them significant health needs in some volatile regions in the LMIC where your health project wants to operate before it gives governmental approval. It is of utmost importance to make stakeholders, particularly the project donors, confident about your project, especially if you approach them with alterations in the project direction or scope midway in the project life. Respect for the team members and external stakeholders including the donor and government officials is extremely vital if you wish for them to respect and support your leadership. Experiment with, and then learn and practice the effective ways to motivate others even while you manage your health project. This will get you closer to your end goal of contributing to the growth of all those that look up to you for guidance and leadership.

Demonstrating integrity

Honesty and integrity are the hallmarks of ethical management practices. A PM with high ethical values will promote team members based on performance, not on personal relationships, and will ensure diverse members of the project team receive career opportunities and advancements they merit; no one in the team should misuse their power to influence the career growth of others, nor use unethical means to promote themselves and their own careers, to give a couple of examples.

When it comes to project success, an experienced PM knows that every project has flaws. They learn that not everything will run according to plan, and they anticipate mistakes in project operations. Nevertheless, solid PMs with strong integrity do not hide their blunders. They always accept responsibility when things go wrong and learn from their errors. This is integrity, which President Eisenhower characterized as *"...unquestionably the supreme quality for leadership."*

When you take ownership for your decisions and actions that prove to be incorrect, you send a strong positive message to your teammates and set an example for them to follow. And you inculcate in yourself this profound quality that is necessary for becoming a true leader.

Embracing change

Albert Einstein once said, *"The measure of intelligence is the ability to change."* As was the case in his day, in today's world, change is inevitable in project management and personal life. Things that were standard in the past are no longer accepted now. New approaches have emerged and will continue to emerge in global health project management, especially following the COVID-19 pandemic. For example, the PM can no longer expect all team members to gather in the office for project meetings every time. They will need to adapt to hybrid or remote models of management and supervision. Climate change and artificial intelligence are influencing global health strategies and initiatives in LMICs. Highly effective PMs understand such changes and embrace them. If you adopt innovations and transformations quickly and without resistance, you demonstrate the potential of successful leadership in you.

Commanding respect

A PM must earn respect from others. If you are new to project management, this will take time, and you will not be able to always please everyone. However, by working hard at becoming an effective communicator, focusing on stakeholder needs, and maintaining integrity along with the other qualities of leadership, you will earn the reputation of being a respected leader. When you command such respect, you will find it easier to manage your project team and impact professional growth in others.

Being on guard

As you prepare to assume your PM role, you should become aware you will always be on center stage. You will be the subject of discussion in all types of social settings. Some conversations will be positive, but others may prove to be disparaging. You will, of course constantly create and maintain a positive impression about yourself, but you also must recognize that despite all your efforts, some individuals in your team will resent you and can challenge your leadership at any time. There are numerous reasons for this. Some people are divisive by nature, others are jealous of your position, and some do not usually cope well with any authority. These are realities that one must accept and constantly guard against dissatisfied team members that may try to undermine your leadership. Dealing with such individuals early on with decisiveness is necessary to prevent them from causing harm to your reputation, dampening the excitement of other team members, and ultimately hindering the progress of your project.

Being optimistic

Helen Keller defined optimism as *"the faith that leads to achievement. Nothing can be done without hope and confidence."* Optimism is to expect positive outcomes even when things go wrong. And things will go wrong on some occasions when you operate a complex project in the area of global health in a resource constraint context in an LMIC. The MOH staff that your project aims to train on healthcare strategies can suddenly go on strike to protest against government policies. The donor might unexpectedly withdraw funding midway in the project cycle. A disease outbreak such as EVD or COVID-19 can abruptly impact your project staffing, causing fear and confusion within your team. In fact, I did experience these three specific situations in my own career, among other depressing setbacks. All these circumstances, however, made me more determined to strive toward optimism instead of giving up hope.

An optimistic PM looks beyond the crisis they go through and focuses on the actions they will undertake to get the team and the project moving in the right direction. Even when facing disastrous situations, you can develop an optimistic mindset for yourself and the project team you lead. Take care though that your optimism is practical and logical and not based on unrealistic goals or emotion.

Some critical elements for developing an optimistic outlook are to be open-minded and focused on new possibilities, embrace innovative ideas, and encourage teammates to do the same, be proactive and determined, and have confidence in your team as you help them to improve and mature. These are transformative leadership traits that you would want to aim for.

Simple steps to becoming a successful leader

The following steps can elevate you to a high level of successful project management and leadership career. These steps are not exclusive to the global health arena but are applicable in all spheres where individuals perform as managers and leaders. These may pose as a steep climb uphill, but they are manageable steps. However, you will need to work hard at climbing them, as did Mark Zuckerberg, who observed, *"Some people dream of success, while others wake up and work hard at it."*

Commit yourself to your goal

As mentioned at the start of this section, you begin with the end goal in mind. These are challenging but achievable goals that you have set for your career. Now, *commit* yourself to these goals. The motivation to pursue your goals will lead you to success. Each day spend ten minutes reviewing your goals and plans for achieving them. Adjust plans as needed. Having someone in your organization (perhaps a mentor), your family, or your friends circle to hold you accountable to your plans helps you to stay committed.

Remove distractions

List things that divert your attention and takes focus away from your daily priorities. When you concentrate on important things you want to get done, switch off your phone and turn off the television if these distract you from focusing on your goals and prevent you from engaging with what you need to get done. Avoid people that cause stress and connect with only those who positively influence your life.

Become self-dependent

Do not count on others to do the things you need to do to attain your goals. Your best friend cannot sit for an exam in your place. Your roommate cannot go to the gym for you to meet your fitness goal that you set for yourself. Likewise, no one in your organization or project team can do what you must accomplish yourself. You must get in the habit of executing your own plan to achieve your goals.

Modify your plans and perspectives

As you keep moving from one step to the next, you may face challenges and sometimes a few setbacks. Review your plans for attaining your goals and your perspectives. You may need to make adjustments to circumvent or deal with a difficult situation. Take a bit of time to rethink your plans and adopt new perspectives for coping with challenges, but do not give up.

Cultivate a positive attitude

As you have seen in Chapter 1, one must nurture a positive attitude for personal growth and building up others. Trusting in your own ability to succeed gives you self-confidence, replacing negative thoughts with positive ones. It motivates you to keep taking those steps no matter what difficulties you face along the way.

Avoid burnout

Make your goal and the progress toward achieving it an enjoyable process. Obsessing over your goals and overworking on your journey can become burdensome and cause you to get burned out. Instead of seeing these as mundane chores, view them as exciting things for which you want to work hard. Your attitude should not be that you *have* to, but instead you *want* to move closer to your goals.

Learn from your journey

It is gratifying to achieve goals, but it is also very worthwhile to notice the small triumphs and feats you attain as you proceed on your journey. Learning from these exciting experiences can be quite rewarding. Keeping your goals manageable will keep your journey from becoming too laborious. You must be enthusiastic about your goals and the steps you take to reach them. Your enthusiasm will give you a positive and fun experience as you travel the course to leadership maturity.

I hope this advice will help you to not only become well-prepared and emerge as an ideal PM of your project but also develop you as an effective leader in global health. As you embark on your career path, I encourage you to take the knowledge and skills you have learned from this book and apply them in the field where the 'rubber meets the road.' I wish you a fulfilling and exciting adventure in managing global health projects and growing into your leadership role!

Give it your best shot and enjoy an adventurous journey!

Global health project management is dynamic in nature. There are constant improvements and changes in response to changes in health needs, policies, and standardizations. If after reading this book you have feedback for the author on how the subsequent editions of the book can be improved, please send these to:

Dr. Paul Robinson using the email address paulrobinson20707@gmail.com. Thank you in advance.

Answers to multiple choice and true or false questions

Chapter 1 Answers to multiple choice questions (Table 1.1)
1 C,   2 E,   3 A,   4 B,   5 D.

Chapter 2 Answers to multiple choice questions (Table 2.1)
1 D,   2 A,   3 B,   4 E,   5 C.

Chapter 3 Answers to multiple choice questions
Q. 5.   5.1.3,   5.2.4,   5.3.2,   5.4.3.

Chapter 4 Answers to multiple choice questions (Table 4.1)
1 F,   2 D,   3 E,   4 A,   5 B,   6 C,   7 G.

Chapter 5 Answers to multiple choice questions
Q. 5.   5.1.1,   5.2.4,   5.3.3,   5.4.4.

Chapter 6 Answers to multiple choice questions (Table 6.1)
1 E,   2 D,   3 F,   4 G,   5 C,   6 A,   7 B.

Chapter 7 Answers to true or false questions (Table 7.2)
1 T,   2 F,   3 F,   4 T,   5 T,   6 F.

Chapter 8 Answers to true or false questions (Table 8.1)
1 T,   2 T,   3 T,   4 F,   5 T,   6 F.

Chapter 9 Answers to true or false questions (Table 9.2)
1 F,   2 T,   3 F,   4 T,   5 T,   6 F.

Chapter 10 Answers to true or false questions (Table 10.1)
1 T,   2 F,   3 F,   4 T,   5 T,   6 F.

Chapter 11 Answers to multiple choice questions (Table 11.2)
1 C,   2 F,   3 E,   4 A,   5 B,   6 D.

Author's suggestions for case study exercises

Chapter 1 The fundamentals of managing global health projects

In general, you may adopt the democratic (participative) style of management with your project team. However, suppose there are two separate sub-teams that focus on the referral of children and the distribution of supplements. In that case, you may also employ an autocratic approach for these two sub-teams since the issues specifically relate to them. To remedy the issues, the first step should be to understand the root causes of the problems. There may be several factors involved in the referrals not taking place as planned and the delay in the supply of the nutrition supplements.

Once you have a good understanding of the causes, you can make decisions and enforce them through the sub-teams. You need not spend time getting everyone's input or securing a consensus among your sub-team members. They will need to comply and follow your instructions. This is the autocratic style of management.

When the situation is corrected, you might like to revert to your usual democratic approach. However, it is important to ensure that the sub-teams receive the necessary training and close monitoring as well as resources and support for functioning well under your democratic management style.

Chapter 2 Building global health project teams

As a new PM of the project team, it is important to take the time to get to know your fellow team members. Show them that you value their opinions and are open to hearing about any concerns they may have. By showing genuine interest and being a supportive listener, you can encourage your team members to be more receptive to your leadership and guidance. This approach will help foster a more open and collaborative environment where everyone can freely share their thoughts and ideas.

Share with the team your vision for the end result of your global health project. What should be achieved when the project ends? Ensure key positions are filled and each team member has a job description and those that need, a job aid, so they can accomplish their responsibilities effectively.

As a team leader, involve your team members in establishing project objectives and priorities. Show appreciation for their good work in public and help them understand the significance of their contribution. Encourage personal development and career advancement opportunities to motivate them further.

It is important to include your team members in the planning and problem-solving process. When conflicts arise within the team, it is best to act as an unbiased mediator and avoid taking sides. Remember that changing human behavior requires time and effort. As a far-sighted PM, it is vital for you to remain patient and persistent with your team leading them toward success.

Chapter 3 Developing detailed activity plans

As the project is in its initial stages and your schedule is occupied with other crucial tasks, it would be advisable to find a specialist, advisor, or consultant either from your organization or a project partner organization to facilitate the DAP workshop and develop the project DAP document. You may be fortunate enough to find multiple facilitators that can lead different workshop sessions.

Regardless of the situation, as the PM, it is essential for you to ensure that the facilitators are experienced and that you and your team members offer them all the support they need to prepare and conduct the workshop sessions. Ultimately, you are responsible for achieving a productive output from the workshop. If you have the expertise, you may consider facilitating a few workshop sessions yourself to assist the external experts.

Chapter 4 Improving project team performance

It is an asset to have Girma on your team as he seems to be genuinely interested in his project work. Since he is already functioning in your team, we assume he has received his initial project orientation and training on his assignments. To help him improve his organization skills, it would be beneficial to have a coach work with Girma.

To ensure that project outputs are completed on time, a coaching arrangement can help Girma prioritize tasks and set up a schedule for his routine activities. This schedule can be tracked over a timeframe of, say, six months to observe Girma's progress in completing his duties on time. As the PM, you could take on the role of coach if you have the necessary skills and time. Alternatively, you could choose someone senior and experienced from your team or outside of it to work with Girma as his coach.

Chapter 5 Supervising project team members

To ensure an objective discussion, focus on the activities rather than personalities. Discuss what was and was not done, rather than how one person feels about the other's intent or attitude.

Throughout the appraisal cycle, ongoing monitoring to gather specific examples and information about your supervisee's performance is useful. Your team member should understand how you selected the scores for the tasks that were supposed to be completed during the appraisal cycle. Emphasize that these scores are not subjective and are not based on personal feelings.

Conducting mini performance appraisals more frequently than the annual appraisal can help avoid any surprises with the scores you give as the supervisor. These mini reviews make the scores more readily acceptable to your supervisee because you both have met periodically throughout the year to discuss performance-related issues.

Encourage your team member to reflect on the scores and be willing to improve performance. Discuss specific ways in which they can improve. As a critical part of supportive supervision, describe how you will provide support to help them improve their performance in the next appraisal cycle.

Chapter 6 Communicating with project team members

Vinod is a good listener and a notetaker. These are strong skills for a PM. Communicating with the 10 direct reports (team members reporting directly to the PM) is relatively easy. Setting up one-on-one meetings with each of these ten teammates at the PM's office would be a good advice for Vinod. If Vinod met with each of these ten team members individually on a rotating basis that would allow all of them to have regular close communication with the PM at the main office.

It may be helpful to suggest to Vinod that he arrange a weekly project status update meeting for his team. Since some team members are located remotely, it will be necessary for him to establish a system for virtual conference calls to connect with everyone. It would be good to orient Vinod on the online platform that you have been using and which your organization has set up for making virtual conference calls.

Ensuring all team members have access to the hardware and software package that will be used for conference calls, and testing the system ahead of the online calls would be excellent advice you can leave with him. It would also be wise for Vinod to consider the best time for these calls, considering different time zones for those joining from other regional offices or headquarters in and outside of India.

In addition to the weekly meetings, Vinod should use the online platform for periodic planning and problem-solving meetings. Formal and detailed communications can be made through email, while informal quick contacts can be made through texting and phone calls.

You may want to suggest that Vinod get creative and organize a fun virtual team building meeting once a month to engage all 135 team members. There are several ways to organize such meetings using online platforms for remote staff.

Encourage Vinod to actively seek feedback and provide feedback on remote and hybrid communication. This will help him adjust and improve his team interactions based on the feedback he receives from his team.

Chapter 7 Interacting with external stakeholders

This case study describes an actual donor funded immunization project in Bangladesh that was operated by an international NGO in close collaboration with the MOH at all levels. Managing this large project as the PM was my early career experience in global health!

Our project team had already established strong working relationships with key officials in the MOH, including the staff of the EPI program that was responsible for immunization activities across the country. We organized meetings at regional and national levels for district and sub-district MOH health managers, who benefitted from our project's innovative supervision and training strategy. They presented this strategy to their superiors in the MOH/EPI office at the national and regional levels. We then arranged field visits for the Director of the EPI office based at the national level along with other senior officials to observe the changes in the communities firsthand. They were impressed with what they saw and returned to their office in the capital, ready to approve the national integration of our project strategy.

Lessons learned: Establish robust relationships with the MOH at every level. Develop innovative strategies and showcase project outcomes. Support government personnel to present and demonstrate how integrating NGO approaches into the government system can be advantageous. Leverage positive connections with higher-ranking MOH officials to gain their support and approval for the adoption of NGO strategies into their own government programs.

Chapter 8 Managing project budgets

If you find yourself in a situation where your project expenses exceed the budget, there are specific steps you can take to control the damage. However, keep in mind that each budget overrun situation is unique, so there is no one-size-fits-all solution.

The first step is to monitor your expenses more frequently. If you were tracking your expenses once every quarter, consider doing it every month instead. This will help you identify any overruns early on, and you can take corrective action immediately.

Next, you need to analyze why your expenses have exceeded the budget. Once you have identified the reasons, take corrective action and while you are doing so, request additional funds from the finance department and senior management. Obtaining approval for additional funds takes time, so it is wise to submit your request as soon as possible.

While waiting for approval, you may need to improve project efficiency by reducing project activities or the volume of services and deliverables. For example, you may decide to postpone staff training or a regional staff retreat.

You can also consider using unused or underused funds from other budget lines to cover any shortfalls. However, before doing so, consult with the finance department experts and senior management to ensure this does not violate any budget policies.

In summary, if you experience a budget overrun, monitor your expenses more frequently, identify the reasons for the excess expenditure, take corrective action, utilize funds from other line items, and request additional funds from the finance department and senior management. Remember to consult with the finance department before moving any funds across budget lines.

Only rarely will a project end, having no issues with BvA variance. The wise PM will put in place the mechanism to detect these issues as early as possible and take prompt action to prevent further harm to the project. These measures will help to quickly pull the project back in line with the budget.

Chapter 9 Monitoring health project activities

One possible solution is to implement remote monitoring. This involves site staff using handheld electronic devices to send photos, video clips, voice messages, and written messages to their supervisors. Although this method is incomplete, it can still provide supervisors with an idea of the project's progress.

To make this work, it is important to plan ahead. Site staff should receive proper equipment, such as smartphones or tablets, before the disaster occurs. They should also receive training on how to use these devices effectively.

Chapter 10 Evaluating health projects

To get started, you can arrange a meeting with your MEAL colleagues to plan out the baseline evaluation activities. You can invite your project team members to join you in this meeting so they can understand their respective responsibilities. During the meeting, ensure that everyone agrees on the number of data collectors to be recruited, their qualifications, and their specific roles.

It is best to recruit data collectors from the same refugee community where the evaluation will take place. They should have a certain level of formal education, so they are able to read and write, follow instructions, and easily interact with members of the community. They must attend all training sessions to prepare themselves for collecting information using questionnaires, checklists, and guidelines.

Senior members of your health project team can work as supervisors of the data collectors. They will oversee and assist with the survey activities to ensure that the work is of high quality. The supervisors must have a higher level of education than the data collectors and should be trained in both data collection and their supervisory roles. If language is a challenge, the project team should consider recruiting a translator to assist the MEAL colleagues during the training of data collectors and supervisors. Alternatively, there may be someone on the project team who can fill this role.

As part of the preparations, your project team members should find and reserve a suitable venue for the training sessions. This could be a spacious room in a hotel or a school building, equipped with all the necessary amenities. Most often the data collectors receive financial compensation for their work, which the project team will arrange. Additionally, the evaluators, supervisors and data collectors will need transportation to the training venue and evaluation sites where data collection will take place. Your project team should organize local transportation for them.

When working with refugees, particularly in places like Cox's Bazaar, the evaluation team should be aware of potential security risks, emergencies, and unpredictable situations that may arise. You and your team must anticipate these possibilities and prepare well to respond adequately to keep the refugees, data collectors, team members, and MEAL colleagues safe during the field work. Taking these precautions will help the evaluation process run smoothly.

Chapter 11 Reporting on project activities

You might like to follow these six steps.

1. Estimate the time needed to analyze site reports, compile and synthesize them, develop all the components, edit, proofread and share with your team members for comments, then finalize, and submit. Allow for about seven business days, as an example, to complete these tasks.
2. Establish a system with all your site managers for you to receive reports from each site at least seven business days before the submission deadline. Enforcing this deadline will provide enough time for you to prepare the report for timely submission.
3. Send reminders to your site managers a few days before their submission date and follow up immediately if there is any delay in their report submission to you.
4. Clearly explain tasks and deadlines to your team members who might support you in developing different sections of your project report. Follow up with them to ensure timely completion.
5. Synchronize your schedule with the finance department/unit colleagues who will prepare the financial section of the report while you compile the technical section.
6. Submit your progress report once it is ready following all the tasks listed under the first step above.

Appendix A: Sample job description

Assistant Project Manager – Ukraine

Organization: XYZ Agency

XYZ Agency is an independent humanitarian organization that assists the victims of natural disasters, armed conflicts and exclusion. Its activities are based on the principles of solidarity, justice, human dignity, equality of rights and opportunities, respect for diversity and coexistence, paying special attention to the most vulnerable people.

Job Title: Assistant Project Manager
Code: ABC-12-345
Duty station: Cherkasy
Starting date: July 1, 2024
Contract duration: 24 months, renewable
Reporting to: Head of Mission, Ukraine
Supervision of: Training Coordinator, Medical Coordinator, Grants & Compliance Manager

General context of the project

Since the war broke out in Ukraine in February 2022, millions of people have fled to the neighboring countries, raising a big concern on how to manage such an immense flux of people. Shortly after the outbreak of the conflict XYZ Agency set up its emergency response in Ukraine in April 2022. Currently the team in Ukraine is operating four health and nutrition projects in the East and South of the country. All XYZ Agency interventions are embedded in a programmatic approach to respond to the multisectoral needs of the conflict affected population, focusing on health and nutrition response serving internally displaced persons (IDPs), their host communities in areas of displacement, and emergency humanitarian assistance in frontline and newly accessible areas. The project portfolio in Ukraine is supported by several donors and XYZ Agency works with two local partners across the project areas.

General function of the position

The Assistant Project Manager is responsible for supporting the Project Manager in the implementation of the project strategy across the project areas and providing technical input to the team.

S/he is also responsible for developing processes and standards within the respective area of responsibility. S/he will oversee the monitoring and evaluation of the project activities across the project areas and s/he is responsible for supporting the development of the portfolio, contributing to donor reporting, and helping the Project Manager in the area of internal and external representation. Ultimately, s/he will be actively engaged in supporting the Project Manager with decision-making, collaborating closely with the Country Office staff and the Senior Management team in Ukraine.

Responsibilities

Supporting project management (55%)

- Guide the program team (Training Coordinator, Medical Coordinator, Grants & Compliance Manager as well as the Community Health Workers and Volunteers) directly or indirectly as appropriate
- Ensure project coordination and coherence across portfolio
- Support project reviews, monitor the delivery of project outputs based on the detailed activity plan
- Support the design of concept notes, proposals and budgets for cost-related activities in coordination with the project team and in line with XYZ Agency and donors' requirements
- Support the Project Manager with timely communication and information flow on project achievements to internal and external stakeholders

Supporting people management (15%)

- Assist the Project Manager to oversee the project team's functions ensuring daily supervision and regular support to maximize efficient performance
- Communicate with the program team on project status, risks and issues in an appropriate and timely manner. Ensure regular and timely communication between project team members
- Monitor the completion of tasks and ensure good performance and record on appropriate systems
- Support the Project Manager to motivate and coach the program team. Communicate Key Performance Indicators (KPIs) to the staffs so that they are aware of the strategic annual plan

- Consistently promote high standards through personal example so that each team member understands the standards and the behaviors expected
- In collaboration with the HR coordinator, support the project team with continuous training and staffs' development. Inspire the team and provide technical expertise

Strategy and vision (10%)

- Together with the Project Manager, Country Director and the Senior Management team, contribute to the development and updating of the country strategy in alignment with the organizational strategies of XYZ Agency.
- Assist the Project Manager to determine, set and deliver goals and objectives for the project team in line with the organization's strategic objectives
- Help develop in collaboration with technical staff of XYZ Agency, high quality project proposals relevant to the health and nutrition needs in the country
- Support the Project Manager identify funding opportunities and build strategic partnerships with potential donors
- Assist the Project Manager to design and roll-out creative and innovative programming, lead assessments for rapid response or scale-up programming in existing or new areas of intervention
- Together with the Project Manager, Country Director and the Head of Operations, create and implement best practice for project management, processes and procedures

Supporting accountability and quality control (10%)

- Support continuous improvement of project quality standards
- Support project development, implementation, ensuring achievements of targets in collaboration with the MEAL department
- Help establish appropriate project management frameworks, systems, and procedures are established and followed, ensuring best practices in project management are developed and adopted

Supporting representation and advocacy (10%)

- Together with the Project Manager, Country Director and Head of Operation, establish strong and effective partnerships with project communities, MOH, organizations, donors and local authorities, in line with the XYZ Agency's country strategy
- Represent XYZ Agency in relevant coordination forums as requested by the Project Manager
- Upon delegation of authority, act as Project Manager when needed

Required profile and experience

Educational requirements

- University degree at Master level in Global Health (MPH) and/or Business Administration (MBA). Advanced degrees in International Affairs, Political Science, Administrative and Financial Management will also be considered.

Professional experience

- Working experience in low- and middle-income countries of at least five years in related activities at Senior Management level is essential
- Experience in coordinating with interdepartmental technical and administrative staffs is essential
- Previous experience with NGOs is essential
- Experience in project planning, budgeting and executing global health strategies is desirable

Professional requirements

- Experience in the implementation of project activities funded by international donors and/or other donors is required
- Sound report writing skills
- Effective interpersonal, communication, and problem-solving skills.

Languages

- English required
- Ukrainian desirable
- Russian desirable

Other requirements

- Computer literacy (MS Office Suite and Internet)
- Organizational skills and ability to meet deadlines
- Teamwork and cooperation
- Negotiation and networking skills
- Cross-cultural understanding and flexibility
- Innovation and creativity
- Excellent budget/financial management skills
- Commitment to XYZ Agency principles

Appendix B: XYZ Agency/Ethiopia detailed activity plan – April 2020 to Sept. 2021

'Immunization for All Children' Project

No.	Activity/Sub-Activity	FY 2020								FY 2021									Status as of 10/15/20 NOTES/POINT PERSON/STATUS
		A	M	J	J	A	S	O	N	D	J	F	M	A	M	J	J	A	S	
1	Improving administration of routine child immunization (RCI) within the Public Sector																			
1.a.	*RCI Implementation in 3 Major Regions*																			
1	[No. 1 above is the activity. No. 1.a. is the target for that activity. Here, in this blank space the DAP gives the sub-activity.]																			[Space is for recording progress with project activities. Project monitoring gives the status information. Useful for progress reporting.]
2																				[This column is sometimes used for indicating the title of the person who is responsible for an activity/sub-activity, or serves as a point person for that activity.]
3																				

Continued on next page

No.	Activity/Sub-Activity	FY 2020									FY 2021									STATUS
		A	M	J	J	A	S	O	N	D	J	F	M	A	M	J	J	A	S	
1.b.	*RCI Expansion to 2 additional Regions and Cities*																			
1																				
2																				
3																				

No.	Activity/Sub-Activity	FY 2020									FY 2021									STATUS
		A	M	J	J	A	S	O	N	D	J	F	M	A	M	J	J	A	S	
2	**Strengthening the monitoring of RCI within the Public Sector**																			
2.a.	*Introduce RCI monitoring tool in 5 regions*																			
1	[No. 2 above is the activity. No. 2.a. is the target for that activity. Here, in this blank space the DAP gives the sub-activity.]																			
2																				

Continued on next page

No.	Activity/Sub-Activity	FY 2020									FY 2021							STATUS
		A	M	J	J	A	S	O	N	D	J	F	M	A	M	J	J	A	S	

2.b. Training of immunizers and cold chain monitors in 3 regions and cities

No.																				
1																				
2																				

No.	Activity/Sub-Activity	FY 2020									FY 2021							STATUS
		A	M	J	J	A	S	O	N	D	J	F	M	A	M	J	J	A	S	

2.c. Supply of vaccine storage equipment to health centers in 5 regions and cities

1																				
2																				
3																				
4																				

Appendix C: Sample staff appraisal form

XYZ Health Organization
Annual Staff Performance Appraisal

STAFF INFORMATION	STAFF OVERALL RATING
Staff's Name:	**Score:**
Position:	
Department:	
Time in this position: ____ year(s) ____month(s)	**O: Outstanding:** Consistently <u>exceeded all</u> requirements of the role.
Evaluation Period: from_____ to_____	**C: Commendable:** Consistently exceeded many of the requirements of the role.
	S: Satisfactory: Performed the requirements of the role adequately.
SUPERVISOR INFORMATION	**RI: Requires Improvement:** Did not consistently meet the requirements of the role. Needs further improvement in performance.
Name:	
Supervised Staff for: ____year(s)____months	**U: Unsatisfactory:** Did not meet the requirements of the role. Did not demonstrate improvement.
Evaluation date:	

INSTRUCTIONS FOR PERFORMANCE APPRAISAL

Performance Objectives and Measures:

Performance Objectives are task related. They are result-based and tied to your day to day task responsibilities as well as special projects. They should be aligned with XYZ's Strategic plan and the Staff's Department Goals/objectives. Three to five performance objectives are recommended.

Key performance measures for each objective. These should respond to the question: how success looks like? Measures can be quantitative or qualitative and should be very clearly defined. Each objective should have one to two measures.

Development Objectives are learning oriented. They are set with the purpose of acquiring or enhancing specific knowledge, skills, or competences (including behavioral competences) so Staffs can perform at a higher level in their current role and/or prepare for new responsibilities in the future. One to two developmental goals are recommended.

SECTION I. PERFORMANCE OBJECTIVES & MEASURES: TECHNICAL

Performance Objectives	Key Performance Indicators/Targets	Ratings		Comments
		Staff	Supervisor	
	• •			
	• •			
	• •			
OVERALL/TOTAL SCORE				

SECTION II. DEVELOPMENT OBJECTIVES: ADMINISTRATIVE AND PERSONAL

Development Objectives	Development Activities	Ratings		Comments
		Staff	Supervisor	

SECTION III. COMMENTS & SIGNATURES

Staff Comments on Self Appraisal	Supervisor Comments on Staff Appraisal
Name:	Name:
Signature:	Signature:
Date:	Date:

By signing, I _____ acknowledge my supervisor and I have met and have discussed my annual performance evaluation.

Index